D1375926

CRITICAL CARE
QUICK GLANCE:
PHYSIOLOGY
AND MANAGEMENT

NOTICE

Medicine is an ever-changing science. As new research and clinical experience broaden our knowledge, changes in treatment and drug therapy are required. The authors and the publisher of this work have checked with sources believed to be reliable in their efforts to provide information that is complete and generally in accord with the standards accepted at the time of publication. However, in view of the possibility of human error or changes in medical sciences, neither the authors nor the publisher nor any other party who has been involved in the preparation or publication of this work warrants that the information contained herein is in every respect accurate or complete, and they disclaim all responsibility for any errors or omissions or for the results obtained from use of the information contained in this work. Readers are encouraged to confirm the information contained herein with other sources. For example and in particular, readers are advised to check the product information sheet included in the package of each drug they plan to administer to be certain that the information contained in this work is accurate and that changes have not been made in the recommended dose or in the contraindications for administration. This recommendation is of particular importance in connection with new or infrequently used drugs.

CRITICAL CARE QUICK GLANCE: PHYSIOLOGY AND MANAGEMENT

WRITTEN BY

Shishir Kumar Maithel, MD

Clinical Fellow in Surgery
Department of Surgery
Beth Israel Deaconess Medical Center
Harvard Medical School
Boston, Massachusetts

EDITED BY

Jonathan F. Critchlow, MD

Assistant Professor of Surgery
Director, Surgical Intensive Care Unit
Department of Surgery
Beth Israel Deaconess Medical Center
Harvard Medical School
Boston, Massachusetts

McGraw-Hill
Medical Publishing Division

*New York / Chicago / San Francisco / Lisbon / London / Madrid / Mexico City
Milan / New Delhi / San Juan / Seoul / Singapore / Sydney / Toronto*

The McGraw·Hill Companies

Critical Care Quick Glance: Physiology and Management

Copyright © 2006 by The McGraw-Hill Companies, Inc. All rights reserved. Printed in the United States of America. Except as permitted under the United States Copyright Act of 1976, no part of this publication may be reproduced or distributed in any form or by any means, or stored in a data base or retrieval system, without the prior written permission of the publisher.

1 2 3 4 5 6 7 8 9 0 DOC/DOC 0 9 8 7 6 5

Set ISBN: 0-07-146540-5
Book ISBN: 0-07-146713-0
Card ISBN: 0-07-146714-9

This book was set in Palantino by Silverchair Science + Communications, Inc.
The editors were Hilarie Surrena, Karen Edmonson, and Penny Linskey.
Project management was provided by Brooke Begin, Silverchair Science + Communications, Inc.
The production supervisor was Catherine H. Saggese.
The book designer was Marsha Cohen.
The cover designer was Aimee Nordin.
The indexer was Betty Hallinger.
RR Donnelley was printer and binder.

This book is printed on acid-free paper.

Cataloging-in-Publication data for this title is on file with the Library of Congress.

CONTENTS

Foreword by Josef E. Fischer, MD / ix
Preface / xi
Acknowledgments / xiii

SECTION I: PHYSIOLOGY

1   Ventricular Function and the Cardiac Output   3
    Abbreviations / 3
    Key Equations / 3
    Factors That Control the Cardiac Output / 4
    Important Pressure and Volume Relationships to Understand / 6
    Differential Diagnosis of Left Ventricular Dysfunction / 10

2   Shock   11
    Abbreviations / 11
    Definition / 11
    Types of Shock / 11
    Response of Organ Systems in Shock / 12
    Three Questions to Answer from the Bedside Examination
        in Determining the Type of Shock / 13
    Treatment of Shock / 13

3   Oxygenation and Ventilation   17
    Abbreviations / 17
    Key Equations / 18
    Oxygenation / 18
    Ventilation / 24

4   Mechanical Ventilation   29
    Abbreviations / 29
    Goals of Mechanical Ventilation / 30
    Basic Lung Volumes / 30
    Indications for Intubation / 30
    Basic Concepts of Mechanical Ventilation and Pulmonary Physiology / 32
    Modes of Positive Pressure Ventilation / 38
    Relationship of Air Flow and Pressure Curves:
        Rationale for Pressure versus Volume Control / 41
    Ventilator Weaning / 42

5   Pulmonary Artery (Swan-Ganz) Catheters   45
    Abbreviations / 45
    Key Equations / 46
    Goals of the Pulmonary Artery (PA) Catheter / 46
    "Normal" Pressures / 46
    "Rule of Fives" / 46
    Waveforms / 47
    Thermodilution Technique for Measuring Cardiac Output / 48
    Pulmonary Capillary Wedge Pressure / 49
    Considerations when Measuring Pulmonary Capillary Wedge Pressure / 49
    Clinical Application of the Pulmonary Artery Catheter / 51

6   Frequently Used Medications: Pressors,   53
    Anti-Hypertensives, Sedatives,
    Paralytics, Blood Products, and Fluids
    Abbreviations / 53
    Receptors and Mechanism of Action / 54
    Pressors and Inotropes / 55
    Anti-Hypertensives / 58
    Analgesics and Sedatives / 60
    Paralytics / 62
    Blood Products / 62
    Intravenous Fluids / 65

7   The Head-Injured Patient: Physiology and Management   67
    of Elevated Intracranial Pressure
    Abbreviations / 67
    Key Equation / 68
    Diagnosing Elevated Intracranial Pressure / 68
    Common Systemic Alterations to Monitor for after Head Injury / 69
    Treatment Algorithm / 71

8   Acid–Base Disorders   79
    Abbreviations / 79
    Key Equations / 79
    Interpreting the Arterial Blood Gas / 80
    Review of the Nephron (the Basics) / 82
    Metabolic Acidosis / 83
    Osmolar Gap / 85
    Metabolic Alkalosis / 87
    Respiratory Acidosis / 89
    Respiratory Alkalosis / 90

9   Nutrition   93
    Abbreviations / 93
    Enteral Nutrition / 93
    Parenteral Nutrition / 99
    Assessing Nutritional Status / 105

10 Prophylaxis Against Deep Venous Thrombosis   107
    and Stress Ulceration
    Abbreviations / 107
    Deep Venous Thrombosis Prophylaxis / 107
    Stress Ulcer Prophylaxis / 110

SECTION II: MANAGEMENT

11 Acute Myocardial Infarction   115
    Abbreviations / 115
    Definition / 115
    Pathophysiology / 115
    Symptoms and Signs / 116
    Diagnosis / 117
    Management / 118

12 Congestive Heart Failure   125
    Abbreviations / 125
    Definition / 125
    Pathophysiology / 126
    Symptoms and Signs / 127
    Diagnosis / 128
    Management / 128

13 Chronic Obstructive Pulmonary Disease Exacerbation 133
    Abbreviations / 133
    Definition / 133
    Pathophysiology / 133
    Symptoms and Signs / 134
    Diagnosis / 134
    Management / 135

14 Community- and Hospital-Acquired Pneumonia   139
    Abbreviations / 139
    Definition / 139
    Pathophysiology / 140
    Symptoms and Signs / 142
    Diagnosis / 142
    Management / 143

15 Sepsis   147
    Abbreviations / 147
    Definition / 147
    Pathophysiology / 148
    Symptoms and Signs / 149
    Diagnosis / 150
    Management / 151

16   Severe Acute Pancreatitis   157
      Abbreviations / 157
      Definition / 157
      Pathophysiology / 158
      Symptoms and Signs / 162
      Diagnosis / 163
      Management / 166

17   Fulminant Hepatic Failure   171
      Abbreviations / 171
      Definition / 171
      Pathophysiology / 172
      Symptoms and Signs / 177
      Diagnosis / 178
      Management / 179

18   Venous Thromboembolism   185
      Abbreviations / 185
      Definition / 185
      Pathophysiology / 186
      Symptoms and Signs / 187
      Diagnosis / 188
      Management / 192

19   Acute Respiratory Distress Syndrome   197
      Abbreviations / 197
      Definition / 197
      Pathophysiology / 198
      Symptoms and Signs / 200
      Diagnosis / 200
      Management / 201

20   Cerebral Vascular Accident (Stroke)   207
      Abbreviations / 207
      Definition / 207
      Pathophysiology / 208
      Symptoms and Signs / 212
      Diagnosis / 213
      Management / 216

      Index / 225

Why another book on critical care? I suppose the best reason is that as patients get more sick, and more and more of them are being cared for in the intensive care unit, certainly in a surgery department, and in a tertiary and quaternary center, it is important that the house staff in particular become familiar with some of the basic tenets of critical care. In many of the existing critical care texts, there is too much of a good thing—that is, too much detail. House officers, and especially practicing surgeons who still take care of very sick patients, do not have the time, patience, or energy to run through a welter of information that contains kernels of truth and kernels of management, pragmatic and otherwise, yet are lost in an enormous amount of detail.

On reviewing this book, one is struck that it is, in fact, both practical and pragmatic. It takes notice of the fact that house officers, young faculty, and young practicing surgeons who take care of critically ill patients have a limited amount of time to read and, therefore, could use a text that is precisely of that nature—that is, a text that is pragmatic and provides necessary and needed information, yet at the same time does not go into too much detail.

Written by two very bright people, Shishir Kumar Maithel, an advanced resident in our program, and Jonathan F. Critchlow, who is not only a superb critical care physician but also an excellent surgeon who is very busy clinically and also technically expert, this volume should be in the case of critical care books, and the necessity to become familiar with it is the best of all possible worlds. For one thing, it deals with the basic physiology of most situations that one is likely to encounter. Second, it is loaded with tables, abbreviations, and introductions to various areas. Third, it provides a brief and pragmatic approach to the therapeutic aspects of situations that one is likely to encounter. Fourth, it does this in a simple, straightforward, and unconvoluted manner with sufficient detail so that the presentation is not "dumbed down" and so that it can be understood.

This text incorporates a rare combination of the pragmatic, the practical, and the theoretical and provides information on a level that is easily understood and can be read with profit in the limited amount of time that is available to any of us.

I have reviewed this text, and write this with enthusiasm. I believe that it will be helpful, certainly to medical students and to junior and senior house officers, but I especially recommend it to young faculty (medical and surgical) and staff, as well as young practicing physicians and surgeons who take care of the very critically ill patients and want to be involved in their management.

Josef E. Fischer, MD
Chairman, Department of Surgery
Surgeon-in-Chief
Chief of Surgery, Beth Israel Deaconess Medical Center
Mallinckrodt Professor of Surgery, Harvard Medical School
Boston, Massachusetts

Critical care management is a skill that is vital to the growing armamentarium of medical students, house officers, fellows, and practicing physicians who take care of very sick patients. However, most texts on critical care are too extensive to read thoroughly, whereas other handbooks on intensive care unit management offer only "cook-book" type instructions to assist with patient care. We feel that it is paramount to understand the theoretical and physiologic basis behind various treatment decisions to deliver the best care to our patients. Written using an outline format, we have included mathematical derivations, tables, graphs, and clinical vignettes to help clearly explain complex concepts of intensive care unit physiology, as well as algorithmic management guidelines for the most common clinical situations encountered in the intensive care unit. Our hope is that this book will be of benefit to all who read it.

Shishir Kumar Maithel, MD
Jonathan F. Critchlow, MD

ACKNOWLEDGMENTS

I would like to sincerely thank Drs. Jesse Hall, Greg Schmidt, and Larry Wood at the University of Chicago, Pritzker School of Medicine, for their incredible instruction in critical care medicine. In Boston, Drs. Larry Gentilello and Ram Nirula pushed me to the next level of understanding the intensive care unit physiology necessary to provide appropriate treatment for patients. Dr. Jonathan Critchlow has continuously provided me with focus and direction. With his unique ability to maintain an extremely busy surgical practice and a strong hand in critical care management and education, he is the model to which I aspire in my own career.

I must also thank my family for all of their support during my endeavors and, of course, Sheetal, who continues to give me perspective and inspiration every day.

Shishir Kumar Maithel, MD

PHYSIOLOGY

To manage patients in the ICU appropriately, it is imperative to understand the physiology that governs an individual's homeostasis. Furthermore, one must appreciate how various diagnostic and treatment modalities reflect and alter that physiology. It is not enough simply to know treatment algorithms for a certain disease state, as patients do not always present in the typical manner. The following ten chapters provide a foundation of knowledge on which each patient's management can be adjusted according to individual needs and clinical situation.

CHAPTER 1

VENTRICULAR FUNCTION AND THE CARDIAC OUTPUT

ABBREVIATIONS

BP: blood pressure
CO: cardiac output
EDV: end diastolic volume
ESV: end systolic volume
HR: heart rate
ICU: intensive care unit
LV: left ventricle
LVEDP: left ventricular end diastolic pressure
LVEDV: left ventricular end diastolic volume
MAP: mean arterial pressure
MI: myocardial infarction
Pms: mean systemic pressure
Pra: right atrial pressure (central venous pressure)
Rvr: resistance to venous return (weighted by volume and flow – stays fairly constant)
SV: stroke volume
SVR: systemic vascular resistance
VR: venous return

KEY EQUATIONS

Ohm's law: Voltage = Current * Resistance (or $V = IR$)

When translated to human physiology: voltage = BP, current = CO, and resistance = SVR

BP = CO * SVR

CO = SV * HR (SV is dependent on preload, contractility, and afterload)

$$SVR = [(MAP - Pra) / CO] * 80$$

$$VR = (Pms - Pra) / Rvr$$

VR = CO (assuming no shunts)

Compliance $= \Delta$ **Volume** $/ \Delta$ **Pressure**

It is important to understand the basic pressure and volume relationships that affect cardiac function and CO to treat patients properly in the ICU. An appreciation for these factors will provide the foundation on which to master more complicated physiology and enable the selection of appropriate therapeutic regimens for patients. First, we examine the central and peripheral factors that contribute to and affect the CO and then graphically depict the important pressure and volume relationships that govern ventricular function.

FACTORS THAT CONTROL THE CARDIAC OUTPUT

Refer to the equations as you work through these pathways.

Central Factors

▶ HR
  • Increased HR decreases EDV.
    ○ Two-thirds of the cardiac cycle is spent in diastole. Thus an increased HR preferentially affects diastole and there is less time to fill the heart. Less time to fill the heart results in a reduced EDV.
      ▪ Decreased EDV lowers Pra.
      ▪ Decreased Pra increases VR.
      ▪ Increased VR increases CO.

Note: HR is not a main determinant of CO, because the effect of increased HR on increasing CO is limited by a decrease in SV ($\uparrow$HR $\rightarrow$ $\downarrow$EDV $\rightarrow$ $\downarrow$SV). Thus, the CO can remain relatively constant over a wide range of HRs. However, if the effect of $\downarrow$SV outweighs the benefit of $\uparrow$HR, the CO can actually decrease (Figure 1-1).

Normal Relationship of HR and CO

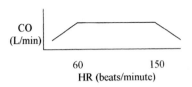

FIGURE 1-1.
CO = HR * SV.

▶ Contractility
  • Increased contractility increases SV.
  • Increased SV decreases ESV.
  • Decreased ESV decreases EDV.
  • Decreased EDV lowers Pra.
  • Decreased Pra increases VR.
  • Increased VR increases CO.

Peripheral Factors

▶ Arteriolar vasoconstriction/vasodilatation (BP = CO * SVR)
  • Vasoconstriction.
    ○ Increases SVR and slightly decreases CO.
      ▪ Thus, overall effect is to increase BP.
  • Vasodilatation.
    ○ Decreases SVR and increases CO.
      ▪ Thus, it can either increase or decrease BP,
        depending on which effect is more substantial.
▶ Venous constriction (70% of the blood volume at any one time
  is in the venous bed; thus, squeezing on the veins will result in
  an increase in pressure) [VR = (Pms – Pra) / Rvr]
  • Increases Pms.
  • Increased Pms increases VR.
  • Increased VR increases CO.

Humoral Factors (Complements Central and Peripheral Factors)

▶ Causes vessel constriction, which increases Pms (leads to
  increased VR)
▶ Increases HR
▶ Increases contractility (leads to increased SV and CO)

Clinical Correlation

A 70-kg young, healthy man is walking down the street with a BP of 120/80, HR 70 beats/min, SV of 70 ml/beat, and thus a CO of approximately 5 L/min. Suddenly, he trips and falls and suffers a severe scalp laceration with profuse bleeding. He quickly loses 1 L of blood (20% of blood volume). However, he arrives in the emergency room with a BP of 120/80. On further monitoring, you see that his HR is 100 beats/min. You quickly realize that his increased HR is compensating for a decreased SV (due to the blood loss) in an effort to preserve the CO. Also, the stress of the situation has elevated his catecholamine levels, which increased his HR and contractility as well as produced peripheral vasoconstriction, which in turn elevates Pms, preserves VR (VR = (Pms − Pra) / Rvr), and thus maintains a relatively normal CO (VR = CO). The SVR also rises due to the vessel constriction. This elevated SVR and a slightly reduced CO maintain the BP in a normal range (BP = CO * SVR). However, this compensation will eventually collapse unless the bleeding is stopped!

IMPORTANT PRESSURE AND VOLUME RELATIONSHIPS TO UNDERSTAND

Cardiac Output as a Factor of Venous Return, Right Atrial Pressure, and Contractility

Note: See Figure 1-2. With normal contractility (solid line), Pra < 5 mmHg is usually sufficient to produce a normal CO (and thus VR) of approximately 5 L/min. However, notice that when contractility is depressed (dotted line), it requires a higher Pra of approximately 10–12 mmHg (i.e., more intravascular volume) to preserve the CO (intersection of dotted lines). The VR is increased in states of depressed contractility due to an increased catecholamine response leading to increased vasoconstriction and, thus, increased Pms.

Clinical Correlation

See Figure 1-2. After a patient has an MI, contractility is usually reduced (dotted curve). At a normal Pra value of 3–5 mmHg, VR is increased (due to catecholamine-driven peripheral vasoconstriction and increased Pms). However, due to the reduced contractility, the curves do not intersect, which leads to a decreased CO and also

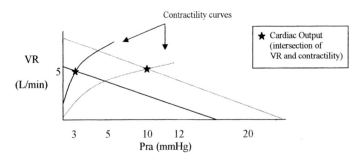

FIGURE 1-2.
CO as a factor of VR, Pra, and contractility [VR = (Pms – Pra) / Rvr].

likely leads to a drop in BP. These patients usually require increased intravascular volume in order to raise their Pra to approximately 10–12 mmHg, thus matching their VR and contractility curves, increasing their CO, and maintaining their BP.

Normal Relationship of Left Ventricular End Diastolic Volume and Left Ventricular End Diastolic Pressure

Note: See Figure 1-3. As the LV fills with blood, a pressure is generated as a function of its compliance. The compliance decreases at higher filling volumes and, thus, the pressure

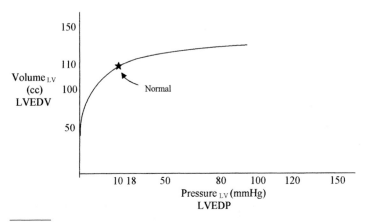

FIGURE 1-3.
Normal relationship of LVEDV and LVEDP.

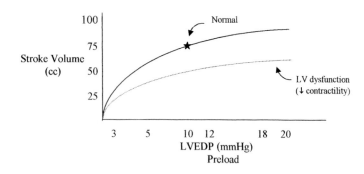

FIGURE 1-4.
The Starling curve.

begins to rise. This decreased compliance observed at high LVEDV is due to pericardial restriction. This limits LVEDV and results in a steep increase in LVEDP. This phenomenon is demonstrated by the asymptotic line (flat portion of the curve) seen on this curve as well as on the Starling curve (see Figure 1-4).

Clinical Correlation
See Figure 1-3. Increasing the LVEDP beyond approximately 18 mmHg has minimal effect on LVEDV and relatively no clinical benefit to the patient. In fact, an excessively high LVEDP can lead to pulmonary edema because the reduced compliance of the LV at such high filling pressures will be unable to accommodate the extra volume, and it can "back up" into the lungs.

Starling Curve

Note: See Figure 1-4. The asymptote of the curve is due to decreased diastolic filling, not worsening systolic function. As mentioned before, diastolic filling is limited by pericardial restriction and reduced LV compliance at high filling pressures. Thus, as LVEDP rises beyond 18 mmHg, there is a negligible increase in SV. LV dysfunction (dotted line) will result in a reduced SV for the same LVEDP compared to normal.

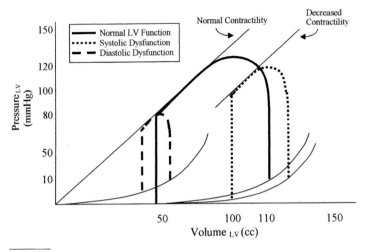

FIGURE 1-5.
Cardiac cycle.

Clinical Correlation
See Figure 1-4. After an MI, any LV dysfunction that follows leads to a reduced SV for the same LVEDP, thus reducing the CO (CO = SV * HR). Increasing the LVEDP to approximately 18 mmHg by increasing the intravascular volume will help to optimize the SV and increase the CO. Once again, LVEDP greatly exceeding 18 mmHg has minimal clinical benefit and may in fact worsen the patient's clinical status.

Cardiac Cycle

Note: See Figure 1-5. The solid line denotes normal cardiac function. Notice that the normal LVEDV is approximately 110 cc, at which point isovolumetric contraction begins. When the LV pressure exceeds that of the aorta, the aortic valve opens and blood empties. The normal systolic pressure achieved is 120 mmHg. As LV pressure falls, eventually the aortic valve closes, the LV relaxes, LV pressure returns to baseline, and the cycle repeats. Pure diastolic dysfunction (dashed line) represents decreased compliance of the LV—i.e., there is a higher LV pressure for the same LVEDV. The decreased systolic pressure generated by the LV is a consequence of its decreased ability to fill with blood; however, it still lies on the normal slope for contractility. Pure systolic dysfunction (dotted line) actually has increased compliance. Although the LVEDV is increased, the pressure generated by the LV is still lower than that of the normal heart, as it lies on a reduced slope for contractility. In reality, most patients with cardiac failure have a combined problem of diastolic and systolic dysfunction.

Clinical Correlation
Imagine a patient with *pure* diastolic dysfunction. A normal LVEDV of 110 cc greatly exceeds the accepted upper limit of 18 mmHg for LVEDP. Thus, these patients need to be *volume restricted* to achieve the desired parameters and avoid pulmonary edema secondary to volume overload and exceedingly high LVEDP.

DIFFERENTIAL DIAGNOSIS OF LEFT VENTRICULAR DYSFUNCTION

▶ Valvular dysfunction
  • Aortic stenosis
  • Mitral regurgitation
▶ Systolic dysfunction
  • MI
  • Iatrogenic (drugs: beta-blockers, calcium channel blockers)
  • Sepsis
  • Hypoxia/ischemia
  • Acidemia
  • Cardiomyopathy
▶ Diastolic dysfunction
  • LV hypertrophy
  • Pericardial tamponade
  • Abdominal tamponade
  • Positive end-expiratory pressure
  • Tension pneumothorax
  • Pulmonary embolism (septum bulges into LV and inhibits filling)
    ○ Right heart syndrome

CHAPTER 2

SHOCK

ABBREVIATIONS

ACE: angiotensin-converting enzyme
BP: blood pressure
CNS: central nervous system
CO: cardiac output
CXR: chest x-ray
HR: heart rate
ICP: intracranial pressure
MI: myocardial infarction

DEFINITION

Shock is a life-threatening condition that results in inadequate end-organ perfusion. It should be differentiated from simply a state of hypotension.

TYPES OF SHOCK

▶ Cardiogenic
  • MI
  • Tamponade
  • Right heart syndrome
▶ Hypovolemic
  • Hemorrhagic
  • Non-hemorrhagic
▶ Septic
  • Infectious
  • Systemic inflammatory response syndrome – noninfectious

▶ Neurogenic
▶ Anaphylactic
▶ Liver failure (sterile endotoxemia – Kupfer cells cannot clear nitric oxide)
▶ Adrenal insufficiency (Addisonian)

RESPONSE OF ORGAN SYSTEMS IN SHOCK

▶ CNS
  • Mental status changes
  • Decreased consciousness
▶ Cardiovascular
  • Hypotension
  • Tachycardia (not a reliable sign – only manifests with > 15% blood volume loss)
  • Cardiac output
    ○ Decreased or increased depending on the etiology of shock
      ▪ Decreased: Cardiogenic, hypovolemic
      ▪ Increased: Septic
▶ Pulmonary
  • Increased respiratory rate
    ○ Results from medullary hypoperfusion of the apneustic center
    ○ Attempted respiratory compensation for a metabolic acidosis (see Chap. 8)
▶ Gastrointestinal
  • Ileus
  • Ischemia
    ○ Example – ischemic colitis
▶ Genitourinary
  • Pre-renal azotemia
    ○ Leads to oliguria (decreased urine output)
    ○ Urine Na < 20, K > 50, SG > 1.020
  • Acute tubular necrosis (ATN)
    ○ Consequence of prolonged renal ischemia/hypoxemia
    ○ Urine Na > 30, SG ≤ 1.010
▶ Skin
  • Cool/clammy (low CO – cardiogenic, hypovolemic)
  • Flushed/warm (high CO – septic)

THREE QUESTIONS TO ANSWER FROM THE BEDSIDE EXAMINATION IN DETERMINING THE TYPE OF SHOCK

1. Is the hypotension due to a decreased CO (Table 2-1)?

TABLE 2-1.
SHOCK DUE TO DECREASED CARDIAC OUTPUT?

Sign	Yes	No
Temperature of extremities	Cool	Warm
Pulse pressure	Narrowed (< 20 mmHg, while normal is 40 mmHg)	Widened
Pulse	Thready	Bounding
Capillary refill (nail beds)	Delayed (> 2 seconds)	Immediate (< 2 seconds)

   If yes – go to question #2
   If no – septic shock until proven otherwise
2. If the patient has a decreased CO, is there evidence of volume overload?
   a. Visible jugular venous distention (**Note:** You can also see this with pericardial tamponade and tension pneumothorax.)
   b. Presence of a gallop rhythm (S3, S4)
   c. Evidence of pulmonary congestion
      ○ Crackles
      ○ Hypoxia
      ○ Interstitial edema on CXR (Kerley B lines)
   If yes – cardiogenic shock
   If no – hypovolemic shock (hemorrhagic vs. non-hemorrhagic)
3. Does something not fit? Do you need more information?
   a. Obtain an echocardiogram.
   b. Place a pulmonary artery catheter (Swan-Ganz) (see Chap. 5).

TREATMENT OF SHOCK

▶ Main principle: optimize rate, rhythm, preload, afterload, and contractility
▶ Cardiogenic
   • Avoid hypervolemia or hypovolemia (but you still need to maintain euvolemia).

- Decrease the preload (maintain Pra approximately 10–12 mmHg).
  - Morphine (causes venous dilatation via a histamine release).
  - Nitroglycerine (causes venous dilatation).
  - Lasix (decreases intravascular volume + causes venous dilatation).
    - Limited by systemic hypotension.
- Decrease the afterload (this therapeutic strategy will be limited by systemic hypotension).
  - ACE inhibitors.
  - Nitroprusside.
  - Morphine (has a slight effect by decreasing pain and thus decreasing the sympathetic efferents and catecholamine response).
- Augment left ventricular function (see Chap. 6).
  - Increase the heart's contractility (maximize inotropy).
  - Increase the HR and maintain it at the high end of the normal range (maximize chronotropy).

► Hypovolemic
- Stop the losses (control any hemorrhage).
- Administer fluids (aggressive volume resuscitation).
- You can use pressors *temporarily* to support the BP while volume is being infused (see Chap. 6).
  - Dictum: Do not squeeze on empty vessels.

► Septic (see Chap. 15)
- Administer broad-spectrum antibiotics and adjust to culture results.
- Administer fluids (aggressive volume resuscitation).
- Pressors (apply peripheral vessel constriction (α effect $\pm$ vasopressin) plus enhance cardiac function (β effect) (see Chap. 6).
- Steroids (if the patient is pressor dependent and adrenally insufficient).
- Consider administering activated protein C.

► Neurogenic
- Administer fluids (maintain euvolemia).
- Pressors (apply mainly peripheral vessel constriction, but you may need to enhance cardiac function because of the

possible bradycardia secondary to a reduced sympathetic output) (see Chap. 6).

▶ Anaphylactic
- Administer fluids (maintain euvolemia).
- Epinephrine.
- Steroids.
- Antihistamines.

▶ Liver failure (see Chap. 17)
- Administer fluids (maintain euvolemia).
- Pressors (same goals as in septic shock).
- Monitor ICP and treat accordingly (see Chap. 7).
- Administer broad-spectrum antibiotics (prophylactic).
- Consider liver transplant.

▶ Adrenal insufficiency
- Administer fluids (maintain euvolemia).
- Pressors (apply mainly peripheral vessel constriction) (see Chap. 6).
- Steroids (Table 2-2).
   ○ Correct the glucocorticoid and mineralocorticoid defect.
   ○ If you use dexamethasone, it will not interfere with a cortisol stimulation test, but it will *not* correct the mineralocorticoid defect.

TABLE 2-2.
EQUIVALENT STEROID DOSES

Dexamethasone	Methylprednisolone	Prednisone	Hydrocortisone
0.75 mg	4 mg	5 mg	20 mg

CHAPTER 3

OXYGENATION AND VENTILATION

ABBREVIATIONS

A-a gradient: alveolar-arterial diffusion gradient
ARDS: acute respiratory distress syndrome
CaO_2: arterial content of oxygen (ml O_2/100 ml blood)
CO: cardiac output
CHF: congestive heart failure
CvO_2: venous content of oxygen (ml O_2/100 ml blood)
DO_2: delivery of oxygen (ml O_2/min)
$FACO_2$: carbon dioxide fraction of alveolar gas
FIO_2: inspired fraction of oxygen
Hgb: hemoglobin
HTN: hypertension
MV: minute ventilation
MVA: alveolar minute ventilation
O_2ER: extraction ratio of oxygen
PaO_2: partial pressure of oxygen (mmHg) – arterial
PAO_2: partial pressure of oxygen (mmHg) – alveolar
$PaCO_2$: partial pressure of carbon dioxide (mmHg) – arterial
$PACO_2$: partial pressure of carbon dioxide (mmHg) – alveolar
PEEP: positive end-expiratory pressure
$PECO_2$: partial pressure of carbon dioxide of expired air
PIO_2: partial pressure of inspired oxygen (mmHg)
Q: perfusion
RR: respiratory rate
RQ: respiratory quotient (VCO_2/VO_2)
SaO_2: arterial oxygen saturation
%sat: saturation of oxygen
SvO_2: venous oxygen saturation
V: ventilation

V_{CO_2}: production of carbon dioxide (ml CO_2/min)
Vd/Vt: dead space
V_{O_2}: consumption of oxygen (ml O_2/min)
Vt: tidal volume

KEY EQUATIONS

$$\underset{\text{O}_2 \text{ bound to Hgb}}{} \qquad \underset{\text{O}_2 \text{ dissolved in blood}}{}$$

$$CaO_2 = (Hgb * 1.34 * \%SaO_2) + (PaO_2 * 0.003)$$

Negligible (except when using hyperbaric O_2)

$$CvO_2 = (Hgb * 1.34 * \%SvO_2) + (PaO_2 * 0.003)$$

Negligible (except when using hyperbaric O_2)

$$PAO_2 = PIO_2 - (PaCO_2 / RQ) \qquad \text{(alveolar gas equation)}$$

$$DO_2 = CO * CaO_2$$

$$VO_2 = (CO * CaO_2) - (VR * CvO_2) \qquad (CO = VR)$$

$$VO_2 = CO (CaO_2 - CvO_2) \qquad \text{(Fick equation)}$$

$$O_2ER = (VO_2 / DO_2) * 100$$

$$MV = Vt * RR$$

OXYGENATION

"Ideal" Blood Gas

  pH = 7.40
  $PaCO_2$ = 40
  PaO_2 = 100
  HCO_3 = 24
  Base excess = 0

It is not only important to know these "ideal" values, but it is also mandatory to understand where these numbers come from and how to derive them to properly use and apply these concepts to diverse clinical situations.

Derivation of Partial Pressure of Oxygen

Atmospheric pressure = 760 mmHg.

Pressure due to addition of **water vapor** by respiratory system = **47 mmHg**.

Assume that atmospheric pressure = 747 mmHg; thus, if you subtract the water vapor pressure, the **dry atmospheric pressure = 700 mmHg**.

Atmospheric air is 21% oxygen; thus, **700 mmHg * 0.21 = 147 mmHg** P_{IO_2}.

However, there is also a **P_{CO_2} of 40 mmHg** in the alveoli (which comes from gas exchange with the blood) that we must account for and that is not part of inspired atmospheric air (remember, the sum of all partial pressures in the alveoli cannot exceed atmospheric pressure).

$$P_{AO_2} = P_{IO_2} - (P_{aCO_2} / RQ) \quad \text{(alveolar gas equation)}$$

Thus, P_{AO_2} = 147 mmHg – (40 mmHg / 1). (Although normal RQ = 0.8, let us assume it equals one.)

$$P_{AO_2} = 107 \text{ mmHg}$$

However, there is also an **A-a gradient** of approximately **7–12 mmHg** because the diffusion of oxygen is not 100% efficient. (A-a gradient increases at higher F_{IO_2} and approaches an upper limit of 30–50 mmHg.)

So, **107 mmHg – 7 mmHg = 100 mmHg P_{aO_2}** (which is the ideal P_{aO_2} measured on a blood gas while breathing room air).

So, **P_{aO_2} = 100 mmHg** (on room air).

Clinical Correlation
A patient is maintained on a ventilator in the ICU. You arrive for morning rounds and see that his P_{aO_2} on the blood gas is 100 mmHg. At first glance, it seems that this patient is oxygenating well. However, you realize that the ventilator is delivering 100% oxygen to the patient. Quickly, you begin to calculate what this patient's P_{aO_2} should be on 100% oxygen:

747 mmHg – 47 mmHg = 700 mmHg (dry atmospheric pressure)

700 mmHg * 1.00 (F_{IO_2}) = 700 mmHg P_{IO_2}

700 mmHg – [40 mmHg (P_{aCO_2}) / 1] = 660 mmHg P_{AO_2}

660 mmHg – 40 mmHg (A-a gradient at 100% F_{IO_2}) = 620 mmHg P_{aO_2}

So, this patient should actually have a PaO$_2$ of 620 mmHg. Thus, although he is maintaining adequate oxygenation, he has a very high A-a gradient, which reflects his severe pulmonary dysfunction.

Oxygen–Disassociation Curve (Relationship of PaO$_2$ and %sat)

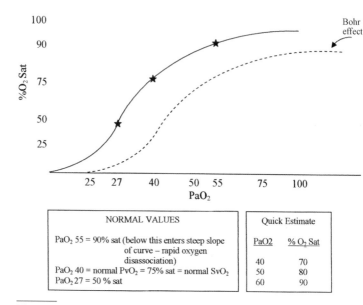

NORMAL VALUES	Quick Estimate	
PaO$_2$ 55 = 90% sat (below this enters steep slope of curve – rapid oxygen disassociation)	PaO2	% O$_2$ Sat
	40	70
PaO$_2$ 40 = normal PvO$_2$ = 75% sat = normal SvO$_2$	50	80
PaO$_2$ 27 = 50 % sat	60	90

FIGURE 3-1.

Oxygen-disassociation curve.

Bohr effect (Figure 3-1): Shifts the curve (dashed line) to the right, which leads to increased oxygen disassociation at the same PaO$_2$, a decreased %sat at the same PaO$_2$, and thus an increased oxygen delivery to peripheral tissues.

Causes of the Bohr effect include:

- Elevated PaCO$_2$
- Increased temperature
- Decreased pH (acidemia)
- Increased 2,3-diphosphoglycerate (2,3 DPG)

Note: Technically, the Bohr effect refers specifically to the effect of elevated PaCO$_2$; however, it is likely mediated by the subsequently decreased pH, and the term is commonly used to include all four factors listed above.

Oxygen Delivery and Consumption

First, let us calculate the CaO_2:

> $CaO_2 = Hgb * 1.34 * \%sat$ (ignore the dissolved component)
>
> Assume Hgb = 15 ml / 100 ml blood
>
> %sat = 100%
>
> 1.34 = constant

Then,

> $CaO_2 = 15 * 1.34 * 1.00 = $ **20 ml O_2/100 ml blood**

Using this value for CaO_2, let us now calculate the ideal DO_2:

> $DO_2 = CO * CaO_2$
>
> Assume CO = 5 L/min = 5000 ml/min (normal value for a 70-kg man)

Then,

> $DO_2 = 5000$ ml/min * 20 ml O_2 / 100 ml blood
>
> $= $ **1000 ml O_2/min**

Now, let us calculate the VO_2:

> $VO_2 = CO * (CaO_2 - CvO_2)$

> $CvO_2 = Hgb * 1.34 * \%sat$
> If: $\qquad$ Hgb = 15
> $\qquad\qquad$ SvO_2 %sat = 75% (normal value)
> Then:
> $CvO_2 = 15 * 1.34 * 0.75$
> $\qquad = 15$ ml O_2/100 ml blood

Then,

> $VO_2 = 5000$ ml/min * [(20 – 15) ml O_2 / 100 ml blood]
>
> $= 250$ ml O_2 / min

Using these values for DO_2 and VO_2, let us calculate the oxygen extraction ratio:

> $O_2ER = (VO_2 / DO_2) * 100$

Thus,

O_2ER = 250 / 1000 * 100

= **25%** (under normal conditions) **(maximal O_2ER is 50%)**

Clinical Correlation

A 70-kg young, healthy male is involved in a motor vehicle crash and arrives in the emergency room. He has sustained significant blood loss and his Hgb is 7.5. His SaO_2 remains 100%, and because he is young and healthy, his heart is able to maintain a cardiac output of 5000 ml/min. You quickly calculate that his CaO_2 is reduced to 10 ml O_2/100 ml blood (7.5 * 1.34 * 1.00), which is half the normal value. Thus, his DO_2 is also reduced to 500 ml O_2/min (5000 ml/min * 10 ml O_2/100 ml blood). To maintain his needed VO_2 of 250 ml O_2/min, you realize that his body must be extracting 50% of the delivered oxygen. You know that he has reached his maximal oxygen extraction capability, and any further blood loss will push him into anaerobic metabolism. Thus, you quickly begin transfusing blood to improve his oxygen carrying capacity and rush him off to the operating room to stop the internal bleeding!

Understanding the Fick Equation [VO_2 = CO * (CaO_2 – CvO_2)]

Normally, VO_2 = 250 ml O_2/min.

250 ml O_2/min = 5000 ml/min [(20 – 15) ml O_2/100 ml blood]

Assume the patient has an MI and CO falls to 2500 ml/min.

The CaO_2 remains constant because Hgb and arterial %sat (SaO_2) have not changed.

Thus,

250 ml O_2/min = 2500 ml/min [(20 – CvO_2) ml O_2/100 ml blood]

To maintain the same VO_2 of 250 ml O_2 / min, the CvO_2 must decrease to 10.

250 ml O_2/min = 2500 ml/min [(20 – 10) ml O_2/100 ml blood]

Remember,

CvO_2 = Hgb * 1.34 * %sat

10 = 15 * 1.34 * %sat

So,

Venous %sat = 50% (SvO_2)

The body compensated for the decrease in CO with an increase in oxygen extraction to maintain the same VO_2. This is manifested as a decrease in SvO_2 from the normal value of 75% to 50%. The maximal oxygen extraction that the body is capable of is 50%. Beyond this, the body is forced to convert to anaerobic metabolism and is predisposed to lactic acidosis. As a clinician, you can use the measured value of the SvO_2 to guide your management. As the SvO_2 approaches 50%, you know that the patient is approaching the limit of oxygen extraction; thus, you must do something to improve the DO_2 or reduce the VO_2.

Treatment Modalities for Delivery of Oxygen/Consumption of Oxygen Mismatch

- Increase DO_2 (delivery)
    1. Increase CO
    2. Increase hemoglobin (transfuse blood)
    3. Increase SaO_2
- Decrease VO_2 (consumption)
    4. Cool the patient
    5. Antipyretics
    6. Sedate the patient
    7. Mechanical ventilation (decreases work of breathing)
    8. Paralyze the patient

Relationship of VO_2 and DO_2 (Figure 3-2)

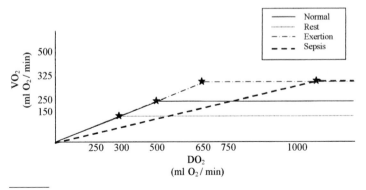

FIGURE 3-2.
Relationship of VO_2 and DO_2.

Slope = Delivery **dependent** V_{O_2}

Asymptote = Delivery **independent** V_{O_2}

Note: Keep patient on the asymptote to avoid anaerobic metabolism.

Right-shifted slope in sepsis is due to a decreased oxygen extraction ability:

- The maximal extraction is no longer 50%.
- It is thought to be due to a decreased activity of pyruvate dehydrogenase, which causes glucose metabolism to use anaerobic glycolysis preferentially and generate lactic acid, as opposed to entering the Krebs cycle and utilizing aerobic metabolism.

VENTILATION

"Ideal" Blood Gas

pH = 7.40
$Paco_2 = 40$
$Pao_2 = 100$
$HCO_3 = 24$
Base excess = 0

Again, you need to understand how these numbers are derived.

Derivation of Partial Pressure of Carbon Dioxide

$$MV = Vt * RR$$

Normal Vt = 6–8 cc/kg; so for a 70-kg man, the Vt is approximately 500 cc.
If the average RR is 12 breaths/min, then
MV = 500 cc * 12 breaths/min = 6 L/min

However, the dead space is ⟵
approximately 1/3 of Vt,
so MVA = 4 L/min (4000 ml/min)

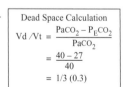

Dead Space Calculation

$$Vd/Vt = \frac{Paco_2 - P_Eco_2}{Paco_2}$$

$$= \frac{40 - 27}{40}$$

$$= 1/3 \ (0.3)$$

Remember, the RQ relates carbon dioxide production to oxygen consumption:

$$RQ = V_{CO_2} / V_{O_2} \text{ (normally equals 0.82)}$$

RQ is affected by dietary intake	
Fat:	RQ = 0.7
Protein:	RQ = 0.8
Carbohydrate:	RQ = 1.0

Again, let us assume RQ = 1. Thus, if V_{O_2} = 250 ml O_2/min, then there is also 250 ml carbon dioxide produced per minute. The carbon dioxide produced in tissues crosses over to the alveoli in order to be exhaled.

Then, the CO_2 fraction of alveolar gas (F_{ACO_2}) is

$$F_{ACO_2} = V_{CO_2} / MV_A$$

$$F_{ACO_2} = 250 \text{ ml} / 4000 \text{ ml} = 0.06 = 6\%$$

To convert F_{ACO_2} to a P_{ACO_2}, we need to multiply by the total pressure in the alveoli, which is 700 mmHg (remember 747 mmHg – 47 mmHg water vapor)

So,

$$P_{ACO_2} = 0.06 * 700 \text{ mmHg} = 40 \text{ mmHg}$$

There is no carbon dioxide inhaled from atmospheric air, so the entire source of this must be from the blood. This explains the P_{aCO_2} on the arterial blood gas of 40 mmHg.

Thus, the normal value of the **P_{aCO_2} = 40 mmHg**.

> **Note:** In clinical practice, the P_{aCO_2} is a *measured* value on the arterial blood gas, and the *total* Vd/Vt of the patient can be *calculated* by using this value and measuring the P_{ECO_2}.

> **Note:** There is a distinction between *anatomic* and *physiologic* dead space, the sum of which comprises the *total* dead space. *Anatomic* dead space includes the upper cartilage-lined airways that do not participate in gas exchange. *Total* dead space can exceed *anatomic* dead space when there is an added *physiologic* component. *Physiologic* dead space can occur in such situations as low CO, pulmonary embolism, pulmonary HTN, or excessive PEEP (which can lower CO and cause capillary collapse – see Chap. 4).

Shunt, Dead Space, and Ventilation/Perfusion Mismatch

These concepts are a function of the relationship between ventilation (V) and perfusion (Q).

$$V/Q$$

Shunt: $V/Q = 0$

A shunt means that there is blood flow (Q) to the alveolus, but there is no air delivered (V). So, blood is pumped past some alveoli without having the opportunity to participate in gas exchange and, thus, is unable to pick up any oxygen. This inability to gather oxygen causes hypoxia and blood desaturation and potentially can reduce DO_2 to the tissues. The PaO_2 falls, but the $PaCO_2$ can remain normal because the remaining ventilated alveoli are still in contact with blood and are able to remove carbon dioxide.

Shunt leads to hypoxia.

Any space-occupying lesion that fills the alveoli can potentially cause shunt. Four main causes are

1. Pus (pneumonia)
2. Blood (intra-alveolar hemorrhage)
3. Edema [cardiogenic failure (CHF) vs. non-cardiogenic (ARDS)]
4. Alveolar collapse

Note: Inhibition of the hypoxic pulmonary vasoconstriction response can also lead to shunt.

Dead Space: $V/Q = Infinite$

Dead space means that there is air flow (V) to the alveolus, but there is no blood flow (Q). So oxygen enters some alveoli, but there is no blood around to pick it up. If there is no blood, those alveoli also cannot remove carbon dioxide and are thus unable to participate in ventilation. This leads to increased dead space and can lead to an increased work of breathing. The $PaCO_2$ rises (due to compromised ventilation and increased dead space), but the PaO_2 can remain normal because blood is still flowing by other alveoli full of oxygen.

Dead space leads to hypercarbia.

Mismatch: $0 < V/Q < 1$ or $1 < V/Q < Infinite$

Ideally, V/Q would be 1 so that V and Q would be equally matched.

However, this is not the case. There are many factors that create the scenario of "mismatch," which is a normal variant of lung physiology. The extremes of mismatch are shunt and dead space. Otherwise, sometimes there is a little more blood flow (Q) and sometimes there is a little more air flow (V). The consequences of this mismatch follow the same pattern of shunt and dead space; specifically, $V/Q < 1$ can reduce PaO_2 and $V/Q > 1$ can increase $PaCO_2$.

West Zones of the Lung

The lung can be divided into three zones, each representing a different relationship between V/Q (Table 3-1):

West zone 1: $V/Q > 1$

West zone 2: $V/Q = 1$

West zone 3: $V/Q < 1$

TABLE 3-1.
ANATOMIC CORRELATION OF WEST ZONES

Position of patient	West zone 1	West zone 2	West zone 3
Standing Supine	Apex of lung Anterior aspect of lung	Middle of lung Middle aspect of lung	Base of lung Posterior aspect of lung

Note: There is a gravitational relationship, as West zone 3 is always "lowest" (Figure 3-3).

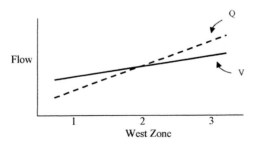

FIGURE 3-3.
V/Q and West zones.

Clinical Correlation

Using this concept, the clinical management of a patient in respiratory distress can be based on specific physiological attributes of the diseased anatomic segment. For example, a patient with ARDS (see Chap. 19) is difficult to oxygenate secondary to a large shunt fraction that develops because of fluid-filled alveoli, which are mostly located in West zone 3. The treatment option of placing the patient in the prone position to improve oxygenation is based on attempting to "reverse" West zones. This reversal can, in effect, convert the less diseased alveoli of West zone 1 to a new West zone 3, thus allowing for more air flow (oxygen) to West zone 3. This change potentially more closely matches air flow (V) to the increased blood flow (Q) that naturally occurs in West zone 3. Thus, this maneuver can potentially reduce the shunt fraction and allow for improved oxygenation.

CHAPTER 4

MECHANICAL VENTILATION

ABBREVIATIONS

A-a: alveolar-arterial
ABG: arterial blood gas
AC: assist control
ARDS: acute respiratory distress syndrome
BiPAP: bi-level positive airway pressure
CHF: congestive heart failure
CMV: continuous mandatory ventilation
CO: cardiac output
COPD: chronic obstructive pulmonary disease
CPAP: continuous positive airway pressure
CXR: chest x-ray
DO_2: delivery of O_2 (ml O_2/min)
ERV: expiratory reserve volume
FIO_2: inspired fraction of oxygen
FRC: functional residual capacity
IC: inspiratory capacity
ICU: intensive care unit
IRV: inspiratory reserve volume
LIP: lower inflection point
Map: mean airway pressure
MV: minute ventilation
PaO_2: partial pressure of oxygen (mmHg) – arterial
PEEP: positive end-expiratory pressure
PIP: peak inspiratory pressure
PS: pressure support
RR: respiratory rate
RV: residual volume
SaO_2: arterial oxygen saturation
TLC: total lung capacity

UIP: upper inflection point
VC: vital capacity (volume of maximal breath)
VR: venous return
Vt: tidal volume

GOALS OF MECHANICAL VENTILATION

- Maintain adequate oxygenation
- Maintain adequate ventilation
- Avoid toxicity and ventilator-induced injury

BASIC LUNG VOLUMES

See Figure 4-1.

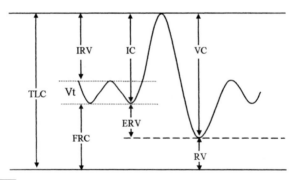

FIGURE 4-1.
Basic lung volumes.

INDICATIONS FOR INTUBATION

Main principle: consider oxygenation, ventilation, airway control, and pulmonary toilet

▶ When in doubt, control the airway.
▶ Intubate if the patient cannot protect his own airway.
▶ Respiratory failure:
  - Type I (hypoxic respiratory failure)
    ○ Increased shunt
      ▪ Pus (pneumonia)

- Blood
- Edema (cardiogenic vs. non-cardiogenic)
- Alveolar collapse
- Type II (ventilatory respiratory failure)
  - Decreased central nervous system drive
  - Neuromuscular disease
    - Guillain-Barré syndrome
    - Amyotrophic lateral sclerosis
    - Polio
    - Botulism
    - Myasthenia gravis
    - Eaton-Lambert syndrome (paraneoplastic syndrome)
    - Polymyositis
    - Rhabdomyolysis
    - Hypokalemia, hypophosphatemia, hypomagnesemia
  - Increased work of breathing
    - COPD (increased total dead space)
    - Status asthmaticus ($\uparrow$ resistance)
    - Interstitial pulmonary fibrosis ($\downarrow$ compliance)
    - Increased elastic pressure of lung
      - Pleural disease
      - Tension pneumothorax
      - Abdominal tamponade
      - Mechanical
        - Severe kyphoscoliosis
        - Severe chest wall edema
  - Increased CO_2 production
    - Fever
    - Sepsis
    - Excessive carbohydrate feeding
- Type III (peri-operative respiratory failure)
  - The problem here is that "closing volume" is greater than the FRC (which is decreased postoperatively), and this leads to atelectasis (discussion to follow).
- Type IV (respiratory failure of shock)
  - Fatigue of respiratory muscles
  - Deconditioning

BASIC CONCEPTS OF MECHANICAL VENTILATION AND PULMONARY PHYSIOLOGY

Closing Volume and Functional Residual Capacity

FRC is the volume of air left in the alveoli at the end of passive expiration. This volume is normally around 50% of TLC.

Closing volume is the volume of air in the alveoli below that alveoli tend to collapse. This volume is normally *less* than the FRC.

Factors that **decrease FRC:**
- Increased age (due to age-related decreased elasticity of alveoli)
- Obesity
- Increased abdominal pressure
- Supine position
- Upper abdominal incision (causes splinting due to pain)
- Hypoventilation in patients with decreased lung compliance

Factors that **increase closing volume:**
- Increased age
- Smoking
- Pulmonary edema
- Supine position

See Figure 4-2.

> **Note:** Usually, FRC is greater than closing volume. You can see that under certain conditions, such as an elderly patient

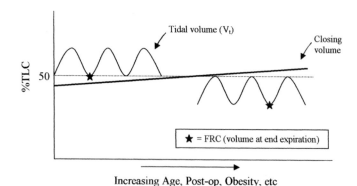

FIGURE 4-2.

Relationship of FRC and closing volume. Post-op, postoperative.

undergoing an operation, the situation can arise in which FRC is actually *below* closing volume. This can lead to alveolar collapse (atelectasis).

Clinical Correlation

A 68-year-old obese female with a 30 pack-year smoking history undergoes a partial gastrectomy through an upper abdominal incision. On postoperative day one, you are called by the nurse because she spikes a temperature to 38.6°C (101.5°F). The patient tells you she is in a lot of pain and is having trouble breathing deeply. You inspect the incision, which looks fine with no evidence of infection. On auscultation, you hear crackles bilaterally at the lung bases. You order a CXR, which shows plate-like atelectasis bilaterally. Quickly, you realize that this patient's alveoli are collapsing because her FRC after each breath has dropped below her closing volume. To remedy the situation and prevent the patient from developing pneumonia, you improve her pain control, order incentive spirometry, sit her upright in a chair, and ambulate her three times that day. On morning rounds the following day, she reports that she feels much better, her lungs sound clear, and her fever is gone.

Note: Preventive strategy for postoperative atelectasis:

- Incentive spirometry
- Chest physical therapy
- Frequent turning in bed
- Pain control
- Early ambulation

Pao$_2$ and Mean Airway Pressure

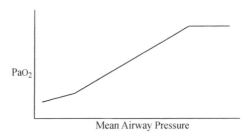

FIGURE 4-3.

Pao$_2$ and Map in the normal lung.

Note: An increase in PaO_2 is positively correlated with an increase in Map (Figure 4-3). This relationship is important when considering different types of mechanical ventilation (see discussion below).

Peak Inspiratory Pressure (PIP) and Plateau (Pause) Pressures

PIP: A measurement of **dynamic** pressure. It reflects **upper airway resistance** to air flow as well as the **intra-alveolar elastic pressure** generated from air entering the alveoli (which is increased by any space-occupying lesion in the alveoli and increased chest wall resistance). However, the PIP will *not* enable differentiation between the two areas of the lung, as it only reports one number as the sum of the two pressures generated.

Plateau pressure: A measurement of **static** pressure. It reflects the pressure generated due to a static column of air. Because the cartilage-lined upper airways do not contribute any elastic pressure, and there is no resistance to a static column of air to generate any pressure (no air flow $\rightarrow$ no resistance), the plateau pressure is a reflection of **intra-alveolar elastic pressure** only. It is measured by instituting a short pause in the respiratory cycle (0.5–1.0 second) on the ventilator at end inspiration.

Using these numbers: The difference between the two measurements, or the **"peak to pause,"** provides valuable information about where the lung pathology lies. If the peak to pause difference is large, it implies that there is increased upper airway resistance (e.g., COPD, asthma exacerbation), and the alveolar elastic pressure is relatively normal. If the peak to pause difference is small, it implies that the upper airways are relatively normal, but there is an increase in alveolar or chest wall elastic pressure (e.g., pneumonia, CHF, chest wall edema).

- Remember, the PIP increases in either situation, whereas the pause pressure only increases with alveolar or chest wall pathology.
- A plateau pressure of > 30–35 cmH_2O places the patient at risk for barotrauma (alveolar rupture). The level of PIP is **not** predictive of barotrauma.

Clinical Correlation

You arrive in the ICU on Monday morning to find two new patients just recently admitted, both of whom are mechanically ventilated. They both arrived in respiratory distress, of which the etiology was unclear. You measure each patient's PIP and plateau pressure on the ventilator (Table 4-1).

TABLE 4-1.
PEAK TO PAUSE PRESSURES, DAY 1

Patient	PIP (cmH$_2$O)	Plateau (cmH$_2$O)	Peak to pause (cmH$_2$O)
1	30	8	22
2	30	25	5

Although they both have the same PIP, you quickly realize that Patient 1 has upper airway constriction as a source of respiratory distress, whereas Patient 2 has alveolar pathology. You administer albuterol and ipratropium bromide (Atrovent) bronchodilator treatment to Patient 1. A CXR of Patient 2 is consistent with CHF and alveolar flooding; thus, you order aggressive diuresis. The following day, you arrive for morning rounds and find the parameters in Table 4-2.

TABLE 4-2.
PEAK TO PAUSE PRESSURES, DAY 2

Patient	PIP (cmH$_2$O)	Plateau (cmH$_2$O)	Peak to pause (cmH$_2$O)
1	18	8	10
2	18	8	10

Both patients are doing much better. Later that day, family members arrive for both patients and inform you that Patient 1 is a severe asthmatic and Patient 2 has a history of CHF and had recently run out of his "water-pill."

Positive End-Expiratory Pressure (PEEP)

- Minimizes cyclic opening and closing of alveoli by keeping alveoli between LIP and UIP, thus reducing shear force on alveoli and minimizing alveolar damage (see Figure 4-4).

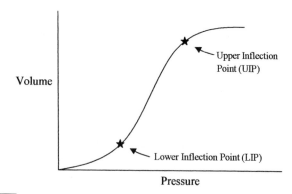

FIGURE 4-4.
Alveolar compliance curve.

- Increases end-expiratory volume (FRC).
- Reduces regional lung overdistention by increasing the number of functional lung units participating in gas exchange and oxygenation.
- Decreases the shunt fraction, thereby improving oxygenation.
- Maintains Map throughout ventilatory cycle, thereby increasing PaO_2 (remember, Map and PaO_2 are positively correlated).
- Can decrease CO in highly compliant lungs by increasing intra-thoracic pressure and, thus, decreasing VR. However, in situations in which high amounts of PEEP are used, the lungs are diseased with low compliance; thus, the pressure does not transmit to the intra-thoracic space. A small amount of physiologic PEEP (5 cmH_2O) does not significantly affect hemodynamics (CO and VR) even in normal, highly compliant lungs.

The goals of PEEP are
1. To optimize oxygenation (SaO_2)
2. To allow usage of a nontoxic FIO_2 ($\leq 50–60\%$)
3. To not diminish overall oxygen delivery (by not causing a significant decrease in CO)
4. To minimize alveolar damage by maintaining the alveoli within the highest compliance portion (steepest slope) of the curve (between LIP and UIP)

Clinical Correlation

A 60-year-old man is mechanically ventilated for ARDS (see Chap. 19). When you arrive in the ICU, you see that he has been oxygenated with 100% FIO_2 for the past 18 hours. His SaO_2 is 90%, and his PaO_2 is only 55 mmHg. Quickly, you realize that he has a large A-a gradient and is not oxygenating well at all. On examination of his ventilator settings, you notice that the PEEP is only set at 5 cmH$_2$O. You begin to increase his level of PEEP and notice that the SaO_2 also begins to rise. Your final settings include a PEEP of 20 cmH$_2$O, and you were able to reduce his FIO_2 to 0.60 (60%). ABG is obtained, which reveals a PaO_2 of 90 mmHg and an SaO_2 of 95%. Because his lungs are so stiff and poorly compliant, his hemodynamics and BP are *not* affected by this high level of PEEP. In fact, the improvement in oxygenation (SaO_2) actually *improves* his DO_2.

AutoPEEP

AutoPEEP is a positive intra-alveolar pressure that develops at end-expiration secondary to incomplete expiration of the total Vt. This creates a positive pressure gradient in the alveoli relative to the proximal airways and atmospheric pressure. This phenomenon is usually seen in obstructive lung disease, such as COPD and asthma. The exact amount of positive pressure generated by autoPEEP can be quantified in a patient who is mechanically ventilated.

Issues of an Increasing AutoPEEP

▶ Increases risk for barotrauma if it causes the plateau pressure to exceed 35 cmH$_2$O (similar to PEEP).
▶ May decrease the CO in highly compliant lungs because the increased pressure can transmit to the intra-thoracic space and decrease VR (similar to PEEP).
▶ Increases the patient's work of breathing:
  • Spontaneous breathing involves the patient creating a negative intra-thoracic pressure relative to atmospheric pressure, which then "pulls" air into the lungs.
  • Normally, when the epiglottis is open, the pressure in the alveoli is equal to atmospheric pressure; thus, there is no pressure gradient.
  • If the patient is unable to exhale the Vt, the trapped alveolar air creates a positive pressure in the alveoli relative to atmospheric pressure.

- • The patient must then generate a greater negative pressure than normal in order to overcome the autoPEEP positive pressure that developed in the alveoli. This increases the work of breathing.
- ▶ Decreases the effective Vt due to a "stacking" of breaths in the airways, thereby increasing the *physiologic* dead space. Remember, increased dead space increases the work of breathing.

Management of a Mechanically Ventilated Patient with Increasing AutoPEEP

- ▶ Decrease Vt
  - • Lowers the volume to exhale
- ▶ Decrease the RR
  - • Allows more time for expiration
- ▶ Increase the inspiratory flow rate
  - • Decreases the time needed for inspiration and allows more time for expiration
- ▶ Apply PEEP to the same level of autoPEEP
  - • Equalizes the autoPEEP positive pressure that developed in the alveoli, thereby equalizing the pressure between the proximal airways and alveoli. By removing the pressure gradient, any spontaneous breaths attempted by the patient will require less work.

Clinical Correlation

A patient with severe COPD suffers from an exacerbation and requires mechanical ventilation. After 12 hours on the ventilator, you notice that his plateau pressures have risen from 8 to 13 cmH_2O. You measure his autoPEEP (a simple maneuver on the ventilator) and find that it is 5 cmH_2O, thus explaining the rise in plateau pressure. You decrease his Vt and RR slightly, making sure that his total MV is still adequate to ventilate him appropriately. When you return later that day to check on him, his plateau pressure once again measures 8 cmH_2O.

MODES OF POSITIVE PRESSURE VENTILATION

Assist Control Ventilation (AC)

See Table 4-3.

TABLE 4-3.
ASSIST CONTROL VENTILATION

RR	Set on ventilator
Vt	Set on ventilator
FIO$_2$	Set on ventilator
PEEP	Set on ventilator
Plateau pressure	Determined by a function of set volume and lung compliance

Note: Each breath will deliver a set Vt. If the patient triggers the ventilator (i.e., breathes over the set RR), the full set Vt will be delivered for every breath. This mode is primarily used in heavily sedated and unresponsive patients.

Synchronized Intermittent Mandatory Ventilation (SIMV)

See Table 4-4.

TABLE 4-4.
SYNCHRONIZED INTERMITTENT MANDATORY VENTILATION

RR	Set on ventilator
Vt	Set on ventilator
FIO$_2$	Set on ventilator
PEEP	Set on ventilator
Inspiratory PS	Set on ventilator
Plateau pressure	Determined by a function of set volume and lung compliance

Note: The set Vt will only be delivered for the number of breaths set on the RR. If the patient breathes over the set RR, the patient will dictate the Vt by generating his own negative inspiratory pressure. These "spontaneous" breaths are assisted by the set inspiratory pressure support. Avoid setting inspiratory PS > 5 cmH$_2$O to avoid creating a "mixed-mode ventilation" picture.

Pressure Support Ventilation (PS)

See Table 4-5.

TABLE 4-5.
PRESSURE SUPPORT VENTILATION

RR	Set by patient
Vt	Determined by patient and a function of inspiratory PS and lung compliance
FIO_2	Set on ventilator
PEEP	Set on ventilator (this mode converts it to CPAP)
Inspiratory PS	Set on ventilator

Note: Each inspired breath is supported with a set amount of positive pressure that is delivered over the time of maximal inspiration until the flow rate drops below threshold. This is in addition to the CPAP that is delivered during the entire respiratory cycle, which maintains open alveoli. When using this mode of ventilation, the amount of PEEP set on the ventilator is actually the amount of CPAP that the patient receives.

Bi-Level Positive Airway Pressure (BiPAP)

See Table 4-6.

TABLE 4-6.
BI-LEVEL POSITIVE AIRWAY PRESSURE

RR	Set by patient
Vt	Determined by patient and a function of inspiratory PS and lung compliance
FIO_2	Set on ventilator
PEEP	Set on ventilator (this mode converts it to CPAP)
Inspiratory PS	Set on ventilator

Note: BiPAP is a noninvasive pressure support ventilation delivered through a tight-fitting mask. Using the term BiPAP implies a nonintubated patient. However, the same mechanical ventilator can be used to institute this mode of ventilation. This mode usually requires an alert and oriented patient to be effective and to avoid pulmonary aspiration.

Pressure Control Ventilation

See Table 4-7.

TABLE 4-7.
PRESSURE CONTROL VENTILATION

RR	Set on ventilator
Vt	Determined by a function of set inspiratory driving pressure and lung compliance
FIO$_2$	Set on ventilator
PEEP	Set on ventilator
Inspiratory driving pressure	Set on ventilator
Plateau pressure	Equals driving pressure + PEEP
Inspiratory and expiratory time (I:E ratio)	Set on ventilator

Note: Pressure control ventilation mode is usually only used with patients who are difficult to oxygenate and have dangerously high plateau pressures (e.g., severe ARDS). It is usually accompanied with sedating and paralyzing the patient. When using this mode, the set driving pressure + PEEP = plateau pressure. This plateau pressure is held constant for the duration of inspiration.

RELATIONSHIP OF AIR FLOW AND PRESSURE CURVES: RATIONALE FOR PRESSURE VERSUS VOLUME CONTROL

The air flow and pressure curves are different for pressure control compared to volume control ventilation. The differences are a result of the unique manner in which the patient is ventilated in each mode. Volume control sets the volume of air delivered and the resultant pressure generated (Map) is a function of lung compliance. Remember, Compliance = Δ Volume/Δ Pressure. Pressure control, conversely, sets the maximum pressure tolerable, and the volume of air delivered is a function of lung compliance. This pressure limit set by the ventilator is held constant for the duration of inspiration (Figure 4-5). Volume control ventilation can use a "square-wave" or a "decelerating-wave" form for air flow delivery. The square-wave is most often used, and thus is depicted below (Figure 4-5). Pressure control always uses a decelerating-wave form for air flow due to its inherent delivery characteristics – specifically, keeping the pressure constant during inspiration. The amount of air flow delivered must decrease during inspiration if the total pressure is to remain constant.

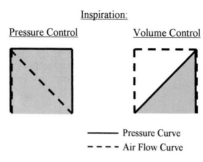

FIGURE 4-5.
PaO_2 and Map in the normal lung.

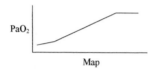

FIGURE 4-6.
Inspiration.

When looking at the figures, it is important to note that the area under the *pressure curve* (shaded area) represents Map, which as you remember, is positively correlated with PaO_2 and oxygenation (Figure 4-6).

Notice that the shaded area under the pressure curve, or Map, for pressure control is *greater* than that for volume control. This increase in Map results in a greater PaO_2, thus offering a greater potential to adequately oxygenate the difficult patient.

VENTILATOR WEANING

Suggested Weaning Criteria: General Guidelines

▶   The initial indication for intubation should be resolving.
▶   Patient is alert and medically/hemodynamically stable.
▶ $PaO_2 > 60$ mmHg on $FIO_2 \leq 0.50$ and PEEP ≤ 5 cmH_2O.
▶   MV requirement is < 10 L/min.

▶ Vital capacity (VC) is ≥ 10–15 ml/kg.
▶ Spontaneous Vt ≥ 5 ml/kg.
▶ Spontaneous RR < 20–25 breaths/min.
▶ Total dead space < 50%.
▶ Negative inspiratory force < –20 cmH$_2$O (more negative is better).
▶ Rapid shallow breathing index (RSBI) < 105.
  • Defined as the spontaneous RR / Vt (L)
  • Also known as the Tobin index
  • Has the greatest predictive value for successful extubation of all the numerical criteria

Ventilator Modes for Weaning

Spontaneous Breathing Trials with a T-Piece or Using Continuous Positive Airway Pressure

▶ Preferred method.
▶ Two-hour trials are sufficient as long as the patient does not fail the trial earlier.
  • Extubation after a successful 2-hour spontaneous breathing trial results in an 18–20% reintubation rate.
    ○ Superior to using "clinical judgment" as a basis for extubation.
  • Success is based on
    ○ No evidence of clinical decompensation.
    ○ Evidence of adequate oxygenation and ventilation as demonstrated by an ABG.
▶ T-piece trial:
  • Patient is disconnected from the ventilator.
  • A T-shaped tube is attached to the endotracheal tube that is used to deliver O$_2$.
  • Patient is monitored closely for clinical decompensation.
    ○ No ventilator alarms will sound because the ventilator is disconnected.
  • ABG is obtained after 2 hours.
▶ CPAP trial:
  • Patient is maintained on the ventilator.
    ○ On the PS mode, the PS is set to 0 cmH$_2$O, and the PEEP is set to 5 cmH$_2$O.
      ▪ This delivers a CPAP of 5 cmH$_2$O.

- Patient is monitored closely for clinical decompensation.
- ABG is obtained after 2 hours.

Note: By maintaining constant intra-alveolar positive pressure, a CPAP trial *may* disguise a patient's predilection for developing hydrostatic pulmonary edema after extubation. On the contrary, a T-piece trial requires the patient to breathe against the added resistance of the endotracheal tube without any assistance, thus facilitating detection of the development of pulmonary edema before extubation. Some providers advocate a T-piece trial over a CPAP trial because it is in effect a "harder" test to pass and, thus, *may* better predict a successful extubation.

Synchronous Intermittent Mandatory Ventilation Wean

▶ The preset RR (which provides full ventilatory needs) on the ventilator is gradually decreased by 2–4 breaths/min every 6–12 hours to allow the patient to take more spontaneous breaths (thereby increasing the work of breathing) until the preset rate is zero.
  - The PS should be set to ≤ 5 cmH$_2$O to avoid mixing the two modes during weaning.
    ○ Patient is monitored closely for clinical decompensation.
    ○ ABG is obtained 1 hour after each ventilator setting change.
▶ Once the preset rate reaches zero, the patient is in effect on PS ventilation with a minimal PS of ≤ 5 cmH$_2$O.
  - A CPAP or T-piece trial can be conducted at this time.

Pressure Support Wean

▶ The amount of PS (which allows the patient to achieve adequate Vt and maintain adequate ventilation) is gradually decreased by 2–5 cmH$_2$O every 6–12 hours to increase the patient's work of breathing.
  - Patient is monitored closely for clinical decompensation.
    ○ RR and Vt are monitored to ensure adequate ventilation.
  - ABG is obtained 1 hour after each ventilator setting change.
▶ Once the PS is ≤ 5 cmH$_2$O, a CPAP or T-piece trial can be conducted.

CHAPTER 5

PULMONARY ARTERY (SWAN-GANZ) CATHETERS

ABBREVIATIONS

BP: blood pressure

BSA: body surface area (m^2)

CaO_2: arterial content of oxygen (ml O_2/100 ml blood)

CI: cardiac index (L/min/m^2)

CO: cardiac output

CvO_2: venous content of oxygen (ml O_2/100 ml blood)

CVP: central venous pressure

DO_2: delivery of oxygen

HR: heart rate

ICU: intensive care unit

MAP: mean arterial pressure

MvO_2: mixed venous oxygen saturation

O_2ER: extraction ratio of oxygen

LA: left atrium

LV: left ventricle

LVEDP: left ventricular end diastolic pressure

P_A: alveolar pressure

PA: pulmonary artery

Pa: pulmonary artery pressure

Pc: pulmonary capillary pressure

PCWP: pulmonary capillary wedge pressure

PEEP: positive end-expiratory pressure

RA: right atrium

RV: right ventricle

SVI: stroke volume index

SVR: systemic vascular resistance

VO_2: consumption of oxygen (ml O_2/min)

KEY EQUATIONS

$$SVR = \frac{MAP - CVP}{CO} * 80$$

$$CI = CO/BSA(L/min/m^2)$$

GOALS OF THE PULMONARY ARTERY (PA) CATHETER

1. Aid in clinical diagnosis
2. Augment goal-directed clinical management

"NORMAL" PRESSURES

See Table 5-1.

TABLE 5-1.
NORMAL PRESSURES

Parameter	Normal values (mmHg)
CVP	0–4
Right atrium	0–4
Right ventricle	15–30/0–4
Pulmonary artery	15–30/6–12
PCWP	6–12

"RULE OF FIVES"

See Table 5-2.

TABLE 5-2.
RULE OF FIVES

Parameter	Pressure (mmHg)
CVP	5
RA	5
RV	20/5
PA	20/10
PCWP	10
LV	120/10
Aorta	120/80

Note: Chambers that are not separated by a closed heart valve should have the same pressure because they will equilibrate with each other. If we examine the cardiopulmonary circuit starting from the right heart, the RA pressure is the same as the RV diastolic pressure (via an open tricuspid valve), much the same way that the RV and PA systolic pressures are equal (via an open pulmonic valve). In the same manner, the PCWP measures LA pressure, which estimates LVEDP because theses areas are all in direct communication during diastole. LV systolic pressure is the same as the measured systolic pressure in the patient (via an open aortic valve). The observed increase in PA and aortic diastolic pressures compared to RV and LV diastolic pressures, respectively, is a function of the pressure created by the arterial elastic recoil against the ejected blood volume in the PA and aorta.

WAVEFORMS

See Figures 5-1 and 5-2.

CVP Waveform

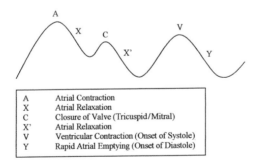

A	Atrial Contraction
X	Atrial Relaxation
C	Closure of Valve (Tricuspid/Mitral)
X'	Atrial Relaxation
V	Ventricular Contraction (Onset of Systole)
Y	Rapid Atrial Emptying (Onset of Diastole)

FIGURE 5-1.
CVP waveform.

Waveform of the "Floating Swan"

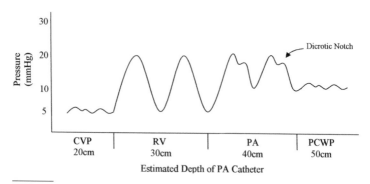

FIGURE 5-2.

Waveform of the "floating swan."

THERMODILUTION TECHNIQUE FOR MEASURING CARDIAC OUTPUT

Five to 10 cc of 0.9% NS at room temperature (no need for iced solution) is injected over 5 seconds in the proximal port of the PA catheter. A thermistor at the distal end of the catheter measures the temperature of the injectate and blood and plots a temperature-time curve over the time it takes for the injectate temperature to equalize with that of blood.

The area under the curve is inversely related to the flow rate in the PA. The longer the time it takes to equilibrate the temperature, the greater the area under the curve, the lower the flow rate in the PA, and thus the lower the CO.

Low COs produce a high and wide curve:

High COs produce a low and narrow curve:

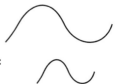

Potential Errors in Cardiac Output Measurement by Thermodilution Technique

See Table 5-3.

TABLE 5-3.
ERRORS IN CARDIAC OUTPUT MEASUREMENT BY THERMODILUTION

Condition	CO
Tricuspid insufficiency	Underestimates
Right-to-left shunt	Overestimates
Left-to-right shunt	Overestimates
Catheter thrombus	Underestimates

Note: In these situations of possible error, one can measure the CO using the Fick equation (see Chap. 3) which uses a nomogram for assigning a standardized VO_2 to a patient based on clinical status and individual characteristics:

$$VO_2 = CO\ (CaO_2 - CvO_2).$$

PULMONARY CAPILLARY WEDGE PRESSURE

When the balloon at the end of the catheter is inflated, it occludes the vessel, thus forming a static column of blood between the catheter tip and the LA. This allows the pressures at the two ends of the column to equilibrate. The capillary pressure measured at the end of the PA catheter should thus equal the pressure in the LA, which should estimate LVEDP (via an open mitral valve). Remember, LVEDP is an estimate of LV end diastolic volume, which is the best estimate of preload. Thus, **PCWP is an estimate of preload.**

Note: PCWP is often used to assess the volume status of a patient (see Chap. 1). A PCWP of 18 mmHg usually implies that the patient is adequately volume resuscitated, and further fluid administration could lead to pulmonary edema.

CONSIDERATIONS WHEN MEASURING PULMONARY CAPILLARY WEDGE PRESSURE

Lung Zones

See Table 5-4.

TABLE 5-4.
LUNG ZONES

Zone	Pressure relationships
1	PA > Pa > Pc
2	Pa > PA > Pc
3	Pa > Pc > PA

Note: PCWP must be measured in zone 3 (Pc > PA); otherwise, the wedge pressure will actually be measuring alveolar pressure. Luckily, PA catheters usually direct themselves into zone 3 because of the increased blood flow due to gravity in zone 3.

Respiratory Variation

▶ PCWP should be measured when thoracic pressure equals atmospheric pressure, which occurs at **end expiration.** End expiration refers to a different point on the tracing depending on whether the patient is being mechanically ventilated or is spontaneously breathing (Figure 5-3).
- Mechanical ventilation (positive pressure ventilation)
    ○ Measure PCWP at the lowest point on the tracing.
- Spontaneous ventilation (negative pressure ventilation)
    ○ Measure PCWP at the highest point on the tracing.

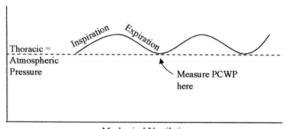

Mechanical Ventilation
(positive-pressure ventilation)

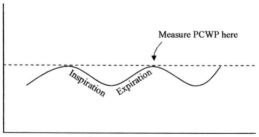

Spontaneous Ventilation
(negative-pressure ventilation)

FIGURE 5-3.

Respiratory variation and measuring PCWP.

Positive End-Expiratory Pressure and AutoPEEP

▶ Either extrinsic PEEP set on a ventilator or intrinsic autoPEEP can affect PCWP measurements because they both prevent the alveolar end-expiratory pressure from returning to zero.

▶ The influence of PEEP and AutoPEEP on PCWP measurement depends on lung compliance, because it dictates how much pressure is transmitted to the thoracic space.
   • High compliance (healthy lungs)
      ◦ PEEP and AutoPEEP can have a greater effect on PCWP measurement.
   • Low compliance (diseased lungs)
      ◦ PEEP and AutoPEEP have little to no effect on PCWP measurement.

CLINICAL APPLICATION OF THE PULMONARY ARTERY CATHETER

The measured and derived hemodynamic parameters available with the use of a PA catheter can help with **goal-directed** patient treatment. You can direct your resuscitation toward the desired hemodynamic parameters as measured by the PA catheter. The trends in measured values can also help make the appropriate clinical diagnosis.

Common Pulmonary Artery Catheter Measurements

See Table 5-5.

TABLE 5-5.
COMMON PULMONARY ARTERY CATHETER MEASUREMENTS

Parameter	Normal value (indexed to BSA)
CI	2–4 L/min/m^2
SVI	36–48 ml/beat/m^2
SVR index	1200–2500 dyne·sec/cm^5/m^2
Pulmonary vascular resistance index	80–240 dyne·sec/cm^5/m^2
DO$_2$ index	500–600 ml/min/m^2
VO$_2$ index	110–160 ml/min/m^2
O$_2$ER	22–32%
MvO$_2$	65–75%

Note: The above normal values are indexed to body surface area (BSA).

Parameter Trends in Various Conditions

See Table 5-6.

TABLE 5-6.
PARAMETER TRENDS

Condition	CVP	RV	PA	PCWP	CI	SVR index	O₂ER	Mvo₂
Hypovolemia	↓	↓	↓	↓	↓	↑	↑	↓
LV infarct	↑	↑	↑	↑	↓	↑	↑	↓
RV infarct	↑	–↓	–↓	–↓	↓	↑	↑	↓
Cardiac tamponade	See equalization of pressures; for example: 20 x/20 x/20 20				↓	↑	↑	↓
Pulmonary embolism	↑	↑	↑	–↓	↓	↑	↑	↓
Sepsis	↓	↓	↓	↓	↑	↓	↓	↑
Liver failure	↓	↓	↓	↓	↑	↓	↓	↑

Clinical Correlation

A 78-year-old female with no significant history of heart disease arrives in the emergency room with a BP of 70/40 mmHg and an HR of 110 beats/min. She is noted to be febrile to 101.6°F (38.7°C), has an elevated white blood cell count of 13.4, is lethargic, and is minimally responsive. She is quickly admitted to the ICU. Large-bore IV access is obtained and fluid resuscitation is started. A PA catheter is placed and her hemodynamic parameters are noted as shown in Table 5-7.

TABLE 5-7.
HEMODYNAMIC PARAMETERS

CVP	RV	PA	PCWP	CI	SVR index	O₂ER	Mvo₂
3	18/3	18/7	7	4.2	640	18%	82%

These parameters confirm your suspicion that she is in septic shock. Thus, you continue with aggressive fluid resuscitation, administer pressors (see Chap. 6) to support her BP, and start broad-spectrum antibiotics. Her blood, urine, and sputum are cultured, and she is found to have *E. coli* urosepsis.

CHAPTER 6

FREQUENTLY USED MEDICATIONS: PRESSORS, ANTI-HYPERTENSIVES, SEDATIVES, PARALYTICS, BLOOD PRODUCTS, AND FLUIDS

ABBREVIATIONS

ACLS: advanced cardiac life support
BP: blood pressure
cAMP: cyclic adenosine monophosphate
CaO_2: arterial content of oxygen (ml O_2/100 ml blood)
cGMP: cyclic guanosine monophosphate
CO: cardiac output
D_1: dopamine 1 receptor
D_2: dopamine 2 receptor
DIC: disseminated intravascular coagulation
DO_2: delivery of oxygen (ml O_2/min)
FFP: fresh frozen plasma
GABA: γ-aminobutyric acid
Hgb: hemoglobin
HR: heart rate
MI: myocardial infarction
pRBCs: packed red blood cells
SVR: systemic vascular resistance
V/Q: ventilation/perfusion

RECEPTORS AND MECHANISM OF ACTION

Alpha 1 Adrenergic Receptor

▶ The alpha 1 adrenergic receptor (α_1) is located on the post-synaptic membrane (primarily skin and abdominal viscera).
  • **Not** located on coronary or cerebral vessels
▶ Mechanism: G-protein–mediated increase in phospholipase C → increases inositol triphosphate → increases cytoplasmic Ca^{2+}.
▶ Action: Smooth muscle constriction → increases SVR → increases BP.

Alpha 2 Adrenergic Receptor

▶ The alpha 2 adrenergic receptor (α_2) is located on the presynaptic membrane.
▶ Mechanism: Decreases intracellular cAMP → causes feedback inhibition of catecholamine release → decreases catecholamine release.
▶ Action: decreases sympathetic activity → decreases BP.

Beta 1 Receptor

▶ The beta 1 receptor (β_1) is located primarily in the heart.
▶ Mechanism: increases intracellular cAMP levels.
▶ Action
  • Increases cardiac inotropy (increases contractility)
  • Increases cardiac chronotropy (increases heart rate)

Beta 2 Receptor

▶ The beta 2 receptor (β_2) is located primarily in the skeletal muscle vasculature and along bronchioles.
▶ Mechanism: increases intracellular cAMP levels.
▶ Action: smooth muscle relaxation:
  • Decreases SVR → decreases BP
  • Causes bronchiolar smooth muscle relaxation → "opens" airways

Dopamine 1 Receptor

▶ The D_1 is located primarily in the mesenteric and renal vasculature.

▶ Action: Causes vasodilatation → increases splanchnic and renal blood flow.

Dopamine 2 Receptor

▶ The D_2 is located primarily in the mesenteric and renal vasculature.
▶ Action
  • Causes vasodilatation → increases splanchnic and renal blood flow
  • Increases the renal metabolic rate, which can increase renal oxygen demand and consumption

Mu Receptor

▶ The mu receptor (μ) is located primarily in the CNS.
▶ Receptor for opiates.
▶ Mechanism: Causes G-protein–mediated inhibition of adenylate cyclase → decreases intracellular cAMP.
▶ Action
  • Analgesia (pain relief)
  • Anxiolytic (anti-anxiety)

γ-Aminobutyric Acid Receptor

▶ The GABA receptor is located in the CNS – adjacent to receptors for benzodiazepines.
▶ Mechanism: Opens chloride channels → influx of chloride ions → causes hyperpolarization → inhibits firing of action potentials.
▶ Action
  • Anxiolytic
  • Amnestic (inhibits memory formation)

PRESSORS AND INOTROPES

See Table 6-1.

Phenylephrine (Neo-Synephrine)

▶ Receptors activated: α_1
▶ Widespread vasoconstriction → increases BP

TABLE 6-1.
PRESSORS AND INOTROPES

Drug	α_1	β_1 inotropy	β_1 chronotropy	β_2	D_1 and D_2
Phenylephrine (Neo-Synephrine)	++++	None	None	None	None
Epinephrine	++	+++	+++	+++	None
Norepinephrine (Levophed)	++++	+++	++	+	None
Dopamine	+++ (high dose)	+++ (mid-dose)	+++ (mid-dose)	+++ (mid-dose)	++++
Dobutamine	None	++++	++	+++	None
Isoproterenol	None	++++	++++	++++	None
Vasopressin	Widespread vasoconstriction				
Milrinone	Increases inotropy and chronotropy; decreases SVR				

▶ Does **not** affect coronary or cerebral vessels
▶ Dose range: 10–300 µg/min or 0.1–4.0 µg/kg/min

Epinephrine

▶ Receptors activated: $\beta_1 > \beta_2 > \alpha_1$
▶ Widespread vasoconstriction → increases BP
▶ Increases contractility and heart rate (both inotropic and chronotropic effects)
▶ Potentially can decrease SVR via β_2 effect
   • Thus can potentially see widened pulse pressure secondary to greater increase in systolic pressure compared to diastolic pressure
Dose range: 2–20 µg/min or 0.02–0.30 µg/kg/min

Norepinephrine (Levophed)

▶ Receptors activated: $\alpha_1 > \beta_1 > \beta_2$
▶ Widespread vasoconstriction → increases BP
▶ Primarily increases contractility with less effect on heart rate (primarily inotropy)
▶ Minimal β_2 effect
▶ Dose range: 2–20 µg/min or 0.02–0.30 µg/kg/min

Dopamine

- Receptors activated: $\alpha_1, \beta_1, \beta_2, D_1, D_2$
- Dose response curve
  - Low dose ($< 5\,\mu g/kg/min$) – primarily D_1 and D_2 effect
  - Medium dose (5–$10\,\mu g/kg/min$) – see β_1 and β_2 effect
    - Both inotropic and chronotropic effects (increased contractility and heart rate)
    - Less β_2 effect compared to β_1
  - High dose ($> 10\,\mu g/kg/min$) – see α_1 effect
- Dose range: 1–$20\,\mu g/kg/min$
- "Renal dose dopamine"
  - Refers to low dose dopamine intended primarily to improve renal blood flow. It is a controversial concept because of a synchronous increase in the renal metabolic rate, and thus oxygen demand, due to the D_2 receptor effect.
  - Fenoldopam: A medication with primarily D_1 effect without D_2 effect. This offers the potential for increasing renal blood flow without increasing its oxygen demand.

Dobutamine

- Receptors activated: $\beta_1 > \beta_2$ (α_1 at very high doses)
- Synthetic (not endogenously made)
- Primarily increases contractility with less effect on heart rate (primarily inotropy)
  - Preferentially used for post-MI hypotension because increasing contractility (and thus increasing CO and BP) causes less of an increase in oxygen demand than does increasing the heart rate
  - Usually decreases SVR (β_2 effect)
  - Dose range: 3–$20\,\mu g/kg/min$

Isoproterenol (Isuprel)

- Receptors activated: $\beta_1 = \beta_2$
- Increases contractility and heart rate (both inotropy and chronotropy)
- Decreases SVR (β_2 effect)
- Dose range: 2–$8\,\mu g/min$

Vasopressin

- ▶ Widespread vasoconstriction at high doses
- ▶ Dose range
  - Sepsis: 0.02–0.08 units/min (usually use 0.04 units/min)
  - Gastrointestinal bleeding (variceal hemorrhage): 0.2–0.8 units/min, with max 1 unit/min
- ▶ ACLS protocol: 40 units (may repeat once)

Milrinone (Phosphodiesterase Inhibitor, Primacor)

- ▶ Mechanism
  - Cardiac myocytes: Increases cAMP → increases Ca^{2+} → increases contractility → increases cardiac output (also increases HR)
  - Peripheral effect: Increases cGMP (nitric oxide pathway) → causes vasodilatation → decreases SVR → decreases BP
- ▶ Action
  - Increases cardiac output
  - Decreases SVR
- ▶ Dose range: Load 50 µg/kg over 10 minutes then 0.25–0.75 µg/kg/min

ANTI-HYPERTENSIVES

Sodium Nitroprusside (Nipride)

- ▶ Widespread vasodilatation (both arterial and venous smooth muscle relaxation)
- ▶ Monitor for reflex tachycardia
- ▶ Metabolized rapidly (half-life is minutes)
- ▶ Potential for cyanide toxicity (rare) – treat with sodium thiosulfate
- ▶ Potential for worsening pulmonary shunt (dilates vessel → increases flow → decreases V/Q)
- ▶ Dose range: 0.3–5 µg/kg/min

Nitroglycerin

- ▶ Primarily a venous and coronary vessel dilator (minimal arterial effect)
  - Decreases pre-load
  - Not a potent anti-hypertensive

▶ Dose range: 0.1–5.0 μg/kg/min

Labetalol (Normodyne)
▶ Blocks α_1, β_1, and β_2 receptors
▶ Dose range: IV load 20–200 mg, then 1–3 mg/min infusion or 100 mg PO BID (max 2400 mg/day)

Beta-Blockers

β_1 Selective

Metoprolol (Lopressor)
▶ Theoretically avoids side effect of bronchoconstriction by not blocking β_2 receptors
▶ Dose range: 2.5 mg IV q 6 hours to 20 mg IV q 4 hours

Esmolol (Brevibloc)
▶ Advantage of short half-life of 9 minutes
▶ Dose range: 50–200 μg/kg/min

Non-Selective

Propranolol (Inderal)
▶ Dose range: 20 mg PO bid to 100 mg PO bid

Hydralazine
▶ Primarily an arteriolar vasodilator (smooth muscle relaxation).
▶ Monitor for reflex tachycardia.
  • Often used in conjunction with beta-blockers to avoid tachycardia.
▶ Dose range: 10–40 mg IV q 4–6 hours (not a continuous drip).

Clonidine (Catapres)
▶ α_2 receptor agonist
  • Decreases catecholamine release
▶ Decreases agitation (decreases central catecholamine release)
  • Attenuates opiate and alcohol withdrawal syndrome
▶ Dose range
  • Oral: 0.2–2.4 mg/day (given as bid dosing)
  • Transdermal: 0.1–0.3 mg/day (change patch q 3 days – q week)

ANALGESICS AND SEDATIVES

Opioids (Analgesics, Anxiolytics)

▶ Act primarily at mu (μ) receptor.

Note: There is a risk of respiratory depression with opiate administration.

Morphine
▶ Very commonly used.
▶ Hepatic metabolism forms an *active* metabolite, which is renally cleared.
  • This active metabolite can cause opiate toxicity in patients with renal failure.
▶ Dose range: 1–12 mg/hr.

Hydromorphone (Dilaudid)
▶ Hepatic metabolism forms an *inactive* metabolite.
  • Preferentially used in patients with renal failure to prevent narcotic toxicity.
▶ Dose range: 1–4 mg/hr.

Fentanyl
▶ Short half-life (effective for approximately 1 hour)
▶ Dose range: 25–200 μg/hr

Note
▶ Use naloxone (Narcan) for opiate toxicity reversal.
▶ Dose: 0.1–2.0 mg IV slow push.
▶ Start with a low dose and titrate upward to effect.
▶ There is a risk of pulmonary edema with administration of high doses.

Benzodiazepines (Anxiolytics, Amnestics)

▶ Act at receptor *adjacent* to GABA receptor

Note: There is a risk of having a paradoxical effect in elderly patients.

Lorazepam (Ativan)
► Median half-life (10–15 hours)
► Dose range: 0.5–10 mg/hr

Midazolam (Versed)
► Short half-life (1–4 hours)
► Dose range: 1–6 mg/hr

Note
► Use flumazenil for benzodiazepine toxicity reversal.
► Dose: 0.2–3.0 mg IV slow push.
► Start with a low dose and titrate upward to effect.

Propofol (Anxiolytic, Amnestic)

► Lipid based – gets stored in fat (try to use short term, 24–48 hours)
  • Adjust fat content in nutrition when using high doses of propofol.
► Decreases BP (arterial and venous dilator)
► Has a short half life (minutes)
► Dose range: 10–120 µg/kg/min

Dexmedetomidine HCL (Precedex)

► α_2 Receptor agonist
  • Decreases catecholamine release
  • Reduces the need for narcotics
► Has a short half-life (6 minutes)
► Continuous infusion should not exceed 24 hours
► Not necessary to discontinue prior to extubation
  • Can be useful for ventilator weaning in an agitated patient, as it does *not* cause respiratory depression.
► Dose range: IV load 1 µg/kg over 10 minutes then 0.2–0.7 µg/kg/hr

Haloperidol (Haldol)

► Neuroleptic – decreases agitation.
► Mechanism – acts primarily via central D_2 receptor antagonism.
► Monitor the QTC interval (if it elongates > 25% of baseline, it can increase the risk of torsades).

▶ May have α_1 receptor blocking effects.
▶ Dose range: 0.5–5.0 mg PO/IM/IV q 2–6 hours (wide range of dosage).

Note: Avoid over-sedation, which is a very common complication in the ICU. Using **intermittent dosing**, as opposed to constant infusions, is an important strategy to avoid over-sedation.

PARALYTICS

Cisatracurium (Nimbex)

▶ Most common *non*-depolarizing paralytic used in the ICU
▶ Mechanism: Competitive binding at nicotinic receptors, thus preventing acetylcholine binding
  • Reversed with neostigmine administration
▶ Composition is not steroid based
  • Decreased incidence of ICU myopathy compared to other non-depolarizing paralytics
▶ Metabolism via Hoffman degradation (enzymatic degradation)
  • Does not rely on liver or kidney function for metabolism
  • Key principle that favors its use in the ICU
▶ Dose range: Load 0.2 mg/kg, then 0.03–0.3 mg/kg/hr

Vecuronium (Norcuron)

▶ Mostly used for short term paralysis needs
  • Paralysis for rapid sequence intubation
  • Duration of action is approximately 30 minutes
▶ Mechanism: Competitive binding at nicotinic receptors, thus preventing acetylcholine binding
  • Has minimal cardiovascular effects
  • Primarily undergoes hepatic metabolism
  • Reversed with neostigmine administration
▶ Dose range: 0.08–0.10 mg/kg IV bolus

BLOOD PRODUCTS

Packed Red Blood Cells

▶ Indications for transfusion
  • Anemia
    ○ No standardized "cut-off" Hgb for transfusion.

- ○ Data support that an *asymptomatic* patient with a Hgb level of 7–9 g/dl does not necessarily require transfusion.
  - ○ Maintain Hgb above 10 g/dl (hematocrit above 30%) for patients with active cardiac ischemia.
- Tissue hypoxia and hypoperfusion
  - ○ Transfusion increases DO_2 (by increasing Hgb and thus increasing CaO_2).
- Hemorrhagic shock
► Considerations
- Average volume 250–350 cc.
  - ○ Monitor patient's volume status after transfusion.
  - ○ Each unit approximately raises Hgb by 1 g/dl and hematocrit by 3%.
- Citrate is used as an anticoagulant for stored blood.
  - ○ Can develop metabolic alkalosis with massive transfusion as citrate is converted to bicarbonate by liver.
  - ○ Can develop hypocalcemia due to citrate binding of calcium with large volume transfusions.
- Universal donor is blood type O negative.
- Universal acceptor is blood type AB positive.

Platelets

► Indications for transfusion
- Platelets < 10K (even if not bleeding)
- Platelets < 20K for a minor procedure
- Platelets < 50K for a major surgical procedure
- Platelets < 100K for a head injury or neurosurgical procedure
- Bleeding after a procedure or spontaneous bleeding
- DIC
  - ○ Common occurrence after severe trauma
- Should not be used as a volume expander
► Considerations
- Pooled product.
  - ○ Multiple donors for a "pack" of platelets.
- Platelets are usually packed into groups of 4, 5, 8, or 10.
  - ○ Each pack should increase the platelets by 10,000 for each group contained in the pack.
    - ■ A five-pack should increase the platelets by 50K.
- Specialized single donor platelets and leukocyte-reduced platelets are available.

Fresh Frozen Plasma

▶ Indications for transfusion
- Rapid, temporary reversal of coagulopathy.
  - ○ Coumadin overdose
  - ○ Vitamin K deficiency
  - ○ Liver failure
  - ○ Dilutional coagulopathy after massive blood transfusion
  - ○ DIC
- Should not be used as a volume expander.
- Should not be used to correct a single clotting factor deficiency when specific factor concentrates are available.
- Effect is short lasting and efforts should be made to correct underlying problem (e.g., vitamin K deficiency).

▶ Considerations
- Average volume is 200–250 cc.
- Contains all clotting factors, von Willebrand factor, and fibrinogen.
- Transfusion may be associated with fever and chills.
  - ○ Treat symptomatically.
- Universal donor is blood type AB positive (opposite of pRBCs).
- Universal acceptor is blood type O negative (opposite of pRBCs).

Cryoprecipitate

▶ Indications for transfusion
- DIC
- von Willebrand's disease
- Massive hemorrhage with a need for rapid repletion of fibrinogen

▶ Considerations
- 10–15 cc of cryoprecipitate contains all the Factor VIII, fibrinogen, Factor XIII, and von Willebrand factor in 1 unit of FFP.
- Usually a pooled product of 10 units.
  - ○ Average volume is 100 cc, which contains the same amount of fibrinogen as 10 units of FFP, which would be approximately 2.5 L.
  - ○ One pooled bag should increase the fibrinogen by 70 mg/dl.
    - ▪ Very useful for patients with massive hemorrhage in DIC (e.g., trauma).

Factor VIIa (Recombinant Activated Factor VIIa, NovoSeven)

▶ Indications for transfusion
- Uncontrolled bleeding in patients with
  ◦ Hemophilia A
  ◦ Hemophilia B
  ◦ Pre-formed antibodies to other procoagulant proteins
  ◦ Severe trauma
- Considerations
  ◦ Manufactured protein that replicates endogenous factor VII
  ◦ Promotes coagulation by activating the extrinsic pathway
  ◦ May cause an allergic reaction
  ◦ Should be avoided in pregnancy
  ◦ Dose range:
    ▪ 60–120 µg/kg IV bolus over 5 minutes
    ▪ Duration of action is approximately 3 hours

INTRAVENOUS FLUIDS

Crystalloid

▶ See Table 6-2.

TABLE 6-2.
CRYSTALLOID INTRAVENOUS FLUIDS

Type	Sodium (mEq/L)	Potassium (mEq/L)	Calcium (mEq/L)	Chloride (mEq/L)	Lactate (mEq/L)	Osmolarity (mOsm/L)
0.9% normal saline	154	0	0	154	0	308
0.45% normal saline	77	0	0	77	0	154
Lactated Ringer's	130	4	3	109	28	273

Note: Most gastrointestinal losses, third space losses, and bleeding are isotonic and should be replaced with isotonic fluids, such as 0.9% normal saline or lactated Ringer's. Large volume fluid resuscitation should be primarily with lactated Ringer's due to the development of hypernatremic/hyperchloremic metabolic acidosis with normal saline.

Colloid

Albumin
▶ Available solutions
- 5% solution
- 25% solution (salt-pore albumin)
▶ Dose
- 25–100 g IV q 4–8 hours.
- Usually given for a limited period of time (e.g., 3–6 doses).
- Should *not* be used to increase serum albumin levels in a malnourished patient with hypoalbuminemia.

Hetastarch (Hespan)
▶ Available solution:
- 6% solution
▶ Dose
- 500–1000 ml IV infused over approximately 30–60 minutes
- Maximum dose: 20 ml/kg/day
  - Taken up by the reticuloendothelial system of the liver, which limits the total amount of infusion
▶ May interfere with normal platelet function

Dextran (Gentran)
▶ Available solution
- 10% solution
▶ Dose
- 500–1000 ml IV infused over approximately 30–60 minutes
- Maximum dose: 20 ml/kg for the first 24 hours, then 10 ml/kg/day thereafter for a maximum of 5 days
▶ May interfere with normal platelet function
- Can also be used for prevention of thrombosis
  - Rate of infusion can be decreased to infuse over 12–24 hours.

CHAPTER 7

THE HEAD-INJURED PATIENT: PHYSIOLOGY AND MANAGEMENT OF ELEVATED INTRACRANIAL PRESSURE

ABBREVIATIONS

BP: blood pressure
BUN: blood urea nitrogen
CT: computed tomography
CPP: cerebral perfusion pressure
CSF: cerebral spinal fluid
DO_2: delivery of oxygen (ml O_2/min)
EEG: electroencephalogram
FFP: fresh frozen plasma
HR: heart rate
ICU: intensive care unit
INR: international normalized ratio
MAP: mean arterial pressure
MvO_2: mixed venous oxygen saturation
NS: normal saline
O_2ER: extraction ratio of oxygen
PA: pulmonary artery
$PaCO_2$: partial pressure of carbon dioxide (mmHg) – arterial
pRBCs: packed red blood cells
PT: prothrombin time
PTT: partial thromboplastin time
SAH: subarachnoid hemorrhage
SaO_2: arterial oxygen saturation

SjO$_2$: internal jugular venous oxygen saturation
VO$_2$: consumption of oxygen (ml O$_2$/min)

KEY EQUATION

$$CPP = MAP - ICP$$

DIAGNOSING ELEVATED INTRACRANIAL PRESSURE

Clinical Signs

- ▶ Mental status changes
- ▶ Altered pupillary responses
- ▶ Increased muscle tone
- ▶ Hyperreflexia
- ▶ Cushing's triad
  - • Hypertension
  - • Bradycardia
  - • Irregular respirations

Radiographic Evidence

- • Standard imaging is CT.
- • The CT reveals anatomic lesions (e.g., mass, blood, mid-line shift, compression of ventricles, contusion, compression of cisterns).
  - ○ It does not give a numeric value of ICP; however, the images provide a clue as to which patients will *likely* have elevated ICP.

Invasive Intracranial Monitoring

- ▶ Place in patients with Glasgow Coma Scale score ≤ 8 or unresponsive patients with abnormal CT scans.
- ▶ You must correct any coagulopathy prior to placing an invasive monitor.
  - • Keep platelet count > 100,000
  - • Normalize PT/PTT/INR
  - • Keep fibrinogen level > 100 mg/dl
- ▶ Types of ICP monitors
  - • Camino bolt

- ○ Placed at the bedside
- ○ Pressure monitor placed intracranially
- ○ Offers **no** therapeutic value. It is solely a diagnostic tool.
- Intra-ventricular catheter (ventriculostomy)
  - ○ Placed at the bedside
  - ○ Pressure monitor placed in lateral ventricle
  - ○ **Has** therapeutic value
    - ▪ You can drain CSF to decrease the total intracranial volume and potentially decrease ICP.

COMMON SYSTEMIC ALTERATIONS TO MONITOR FOR AFTER HEAD INJURY

Syndrome of Inappropriate Antidiuretic Hormone Secretion (SIADH)

- ► Decreased urine output
- ► Increased urine osmolality
- ► Hyponatremia
- ► Decreased serum osmolality
- ► Urine sodium > 20 mEq/L
- ► Treatment options:
  - Free water restriction
    - ○ In cases of SAH as the etiology of SIADH, avoid hypovolemia and hypotension because these states can induce cerebral vasospasm and increase infarct size (see Chap. 20).
  - Salt repletion
  - 3% NS
    - ○ Important that fluid osmolality is greater than urine osmolality as to avoid worsening hyponatremia
  - Loop diuretics
  - Demeclocycline

Central Diabetes Insipidus

- ► Increased urine output
- ► Decreased urine osmolality
- ► Hypernatremia
- ► Increased serum osmolality

▶ Urine sodium < 20 mEq/L
▶ Treatment options
  • Desmopressin (dDAVP)
  • Thiazide diuretics
  • Nonsteroidal antiinflammatory drugs
    ○ Decreases prostaglandin release and thus decreases afferent arteriolar dilatation
  • Replacement of urine output (cc/cc) with 5% dextrose in water (DSW)

Cerebral Salt Wasting

▶ Most often seen with SAH
▶ Normal to increased urine output
▶ Normal to increased urine osmolality
▶ Hyponatremia
▶ Hypouricemia
▶ Normal to decreased serum osmolality (due to a secondary release of antidiuretic hormone in response to the hypovolemia that ensues with an increased urine output)
▶ Increased urinary sodium excretion
▶ Treatment options:
  • Usually self-limited (3–4 weeks)
  • Salt replacement
    ○ Isotonic fluid replacement (0.9% NS, lactated Ringer's)
    ○ Salt tablets
    ○ Hypertonic saline (3% NS) in severe cases
  • Fludrocortisone (mineralocorticoid)
    ○ Enhances aldosterone effect of sodium retention

Disseminated Intravascular Coagulation

▶ Thromboplastin is released after a head injury and can predispose to developing disseminated intravascular coagulation.
▶ Treatment options (replenish as necessary):
  • pRBCs
  • Platelets
  • Clotting factors (FFP)
  • Fibrinogen (cryoprecipitate)

TREATMENT ALGORITHM

Main Principles

▶ The cranium is a closed space with three main components whose sum of volumes remains constant (Monro-Kellie hypothesis):
  • Brain parenchyma
  • Blood
  • CSF
▶ Avoid hypotension:
  • Can decrease CPP and thus worsen patient outcomes.
▶ Avoid hypoxia:
  • Can decrease cerebral DO_2 and thus also worsen patient outcomes.
▶ The main goal is to maintain adequate perfusion and oxygen delivery to the brain parenchyma *without* causing an increase in ICP, which can increase the risk for brain herniation.
▶ The brain's ability to regulate the cerebral blood flow and ICP over a wide range of systemic BPs is impaired in the injured state.
▶ **Maintain CPP:**
  • CPP = MAP – ICP
    ◦ You can administer pressors to augment the MAP in an effort to preserve the CPP
  • Goal: CPP > 65 mmHg but < 75 mmHg.
  • Keep ICP ≤ 20 mmHg

Note: Normally, cerebral blood flow is regulated over a wide range of systemic BPs. However, during the injured state, this autoregulation is impaired (Figure 7-1). Thus, it is imperative to keep the MAP high enough to maintain a CPP between 65 and 75 mmHg.

Note: Figure 7-2 is an example of a *possible* relationship of CPP, ICP, and MAP in a head-injured patient. Assume an injured patient has an ICP of 20 mmHg. To maintain the CPP between 65 and 75 mmHg, you need to maintain the MAP between 85 and 95 mmHg. However, after a new equilibrium is reached, there is a threshold point of MAP beyond which the ICP can potentially rise with an increasing systemic BP. This occurs because the cranium is a closed space, and an increasing MAP can increase the cerebral

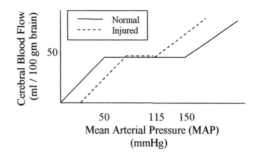

FIGURE 7-1.

Relationship between cerebral blood flow and MAP.

blood flow (remember, autoregulation is impaired), which increases intracranial blood volume, thereby increasing ICP. In this scenario, reducing the systemic BP can sometimes decrease ICP (keeping it ≤ 20 mmHg) while still maintaining an adequate CPP of 65–75 mmHg.

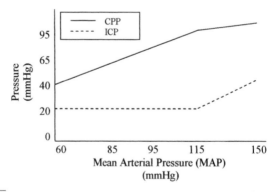

FIGURE 7-2.

CPP and ICP as a function of MAP in the *injured* state.

Head Positioning

▶ Keep the head flat or slightly elevated to 30 degrees.
  • Improves venous drainage, which prevents an increase in ICP due to increasing intracranial blood volume.

► Avoid keeping the patient in the Trendelenburg position for long periods of time (e.g., during central line placement).
  • Trendelenburg position does **not** necessarily augment blood flow to the brain.
    ○ It does **not** necessarily augment *arterial* flow to the brain.
    ○ It can actually reduce cerebral *venous* drainage, and thus can potentially *increase* ICP, thereby compromising cerebral perfusion.

Mannitol

► Mechanism:
  • Osmotic diuresis
    ○ Decreases total blood volume
  • Free radical scavenger
    ○ Can potentially reduce toxic insult to the brain
► You must ensure that the patient is *normotensive* before administering mannitol.
  • Should not be used in the hypotensive patient
► Dose: 25–100 g IV prn.
  • Titrate to effect (no absolute dosing regimen).
  • Endpoints:
    ○ Serum sodium 155 mEq/L
    ○ Serum osmolality 320 mOsm/L

Note: Estimate of serum osmolality = 2(Na) + glucose/18 + BUN/2.8

Fluid Restriction

► Do **not** administer *free water* or *hypotonic* fluids.
► Use *isotonic* fluids (0.9 NS, lactated Ringer's).
  • This potentially avoids fluid shifts into the brain tissue, which can worsen edema and increase ICP.
  • You must be vigilant to mix all meds (e.g., antibiotics, pressors) in isotonic fluids and maximally concentrate them to avoid hypervolemia.
► You must balance between keeping the patient "dry" to avoid worsening brain edema and thus elevating ICP, and under-resuscitating the patient, which can potentially compromise other organ functions (e.g., causing pre-renal azotemia or acute tubular necrosis).

► Trials are under way looking at the benefit of *hypertonic* saline.
  • Theoretically, it can *draw* fluid out of the brain and reduce edema and ICP.

Temperature

► Keep the patient *normothermic*.
  • Avoid hyperthermia.
    ○ Cool the room.
    ○ Administer Tylenol (affects central regulation).
    ○ Apply cooling blankets.
    ○ Apply ice packs (underarms and groin).
  • Hyperthermia can increase cerebral metabolic demands and Vo_2.
  • Trials are under way looking at the benefits of *hypothermia* in cerebral protection.

Glucose

► Keep the patient *normoglycemic*.
  • Avoid hyperglycemia.
    ○ Use an insulin drip or an aggressive insulin sliding scale to keep the serum glucose level between 100 and 120 mg/dl.
    ○ Hyperglycemia has been shown to increase infarct size in the stroke population, and thus can potentially worsen patient outcomes after sustaining a head injury.

Cerebrospinal Fluid

► Drain CSF.
  • If an intraventricular catheter is in place, you can remove CSF and thus decrease the overall volume inside the cranium, which is a closed space.
  • The drain is placed at a height above the tragus, which corresponds to the desired pressure above which CSF is to drain out of the ventricle.
    ○ For example: placing the drain 15 cm above the tragus will cause CSF to drain when ICP > 15 cm H_2O.

Note: 1 mmHg = 1.6 cm H_2O (they are **not** interchangeable)

Hyperventilation

▶ Mechanism of reducing ICP:
  • A decreased $PaCO_2$ causes cerebral vessel constriction.
  • Constriction decreases blood flow to the brain and thus reduces the total volume inside cranium, thereby reducing ICP.
▶ Use only *controlled* hyperventilation
  • Maintain the $PaCO_2$ at 35 mmHg.
  • You must avoid excessive prolonged hyperventilation (e.g., $PaCO_2 < 25$–30 mmHg)
    ○ A new equilibrium is reached within 4–6 hours after which the effect of hyperventilation on cerebral vessel constriction is limited.
    ○ You need to retain this maneuver as an acute *transient* treatment for sudden increases in ICP before more definitive measures can be taken.
    ○ Decreasing the $PaCO_2$ can potentially cause excessive cerebral vessel constriction, thereby reducing cerebral blood flow, limiting DO_2, and potentially making the brain ischemic.

Monitoring Internal Jugular Venous Oxygen Saturation

▶ Principle:
  • Analogous to the MvO_2 measurement on a PA catheter for assessing the relationship of DO_2 and VO_2 in the systemic circulation.
    ○ Remember, the maximal O_2ER is 50%.
    ○ An MvO_2 of $\geq 60\%$ implies an $O_2ER \leq 40\%$ and thus an adequate DO_2 with some margin for error, because the venous blood is returning to the heart at least 60% saturated with oxygen.
      ▪ Similarly, the SjO_2 helps assess the relationship of DO_2 and VO_2 specifically for the *cerebral* circulation.
    ○ Similar to the MvO_2, SjO_2 should be maintained at $\geq 60\%$ but $< 75\%$.
      ▪ This range indicates an adequate cerebral DO_2 but should avoid excessive cerebral blood flow, which can increase ICP.

▶ Monitoring the SjO_2 allows for *goal-directed* therapy:
  • The SjO_2 value can define the limits of hyperventilation as a therapeutic maneuver. An $SjO_2 < 60\%$ implies that the cerebral DO_2 is marginal, likely due to the cerebral vessel constriction induced by hyperventilation. Soon the brain can reach its maximal O_2ER and cerebral VO_2 demands will exceed DO_2 supply. Monitoring SjO_2 is similar to the application of MvO_2 values in assessing the systemic circulation.
  • You should consider using SjO_2 monitoring in the patient with an elevated ICP that is difficult to control and thus requires a certain level of chronic hyperventilation to control ICP. SjO_2 values assist you in determining the ideal target $PaCO_2$.

Sedation

▶ Use heavy sedation in the patient with a difficult to control ICP.
  • Use large doses of narcotics, benzodiazepines, and propofol (see Chap. 6).
▶ Limit external stimulation.
  • Turn off the lights in the room.
  • Minimize noise.
  • Minimize visitors.

Paralysis

▶ If it is still difficult to control the ICP with heavy sedation, you can paralyze the patient.
▶ Cisatracurium (see Chap. 6) is the most often used paralytic in the ICU.

Pentobarbital Coma

▶ If it is still difficult to control the ICP with heavy sedation and paralysis, you can place the patient in a barbiturate coma.
  • Consider this primarily in hemodynamically stable patients, because a pentobarbital coma can cause hemodynamic instability.
  • Wean off pentobarbital as soon as the ICP is < 20 mmHg.

- Titrate the depth of the coma to EEG burst suppression (patient should have continuous EEG monitoring while in a pentobarbital coma).
  - ○ Serum levels do not correlate well with the depth of the coma.

Clinical Correlation

A healthy 30-year-old man is involved in a motor vehicle crash and sustains an isolated closed-head injury. He arrives in the trauma bay with a Glasgow Coma Scale score of 7. He is quickly intubated, IV access is obtained, and *isotonic* fluid resuscitation is started. His vital signs are BP 110/70, HR 75, and 100% SaO_2. A head CT reveals a diffuse intraparenchymal bleed. After arriving in the ICU, you consult the neurosurgical service to place a ventriculostomy drain. In preparation for this procedure, you administer 2 units of FFP to correct his INR of 1.5. Once the intraventricular catheter is placed, his ICP measures 22 mmHg, his MAP is 82 mmHg, and thus his CPP is 60 mmHg. You realize that you need to increase his CPP as well as lower his ICP. His head is appropriately positioned, and he is heavily sedated. You believe that he is euvolemic and thus administer 50 g of mannitol, after which you notice that his ICP decreases to 17 mmHg, raising his CPP to 65 mmHg. His ventriculostomy drain is also placed appropriately to drain CSF when his ICP is > 17 mmHg.

The next morning, his ICP begins to rise and reaches 25 mmHg. You decide to paralyze him, but this only decreases his ICP to 24 mmHg. His serum osmolality is already 320 mOsm/L, and his serum sodium is 155 mEq/L, so you cannot give more mannitol. His $PaCO_2$ is 40 mmHg, so to decrease his ICP, you decide to hyperventilate him and lower his $PaCO_2$ to 35 mmHg. This maneuver lowers his ICP to 21 mmHg. This therapy seems to work; however, you are concerned about cerebral vasoconstriction. You place a catheter for SjO_2 monitoring to help guide your hyperventilation therapy. His SjO_2 reads 70%. Thus, you continue to hyperventilate him to a $PaCO_2$ of 30 mmHg, after which the SjO_2 reads 60% and his ICP is now 18 mmHg. At this time, his MAP is 85 mmHg; thus, his CPP is 67 mmHg. Over the next week, he slowly improves, his ICP begins to decrease as his cerebral edema resolves, and eventually he "wakes up" with intact neurologic function.

CHAPTER 8

ACID–BASE DISORDERS

ABBREVIATIONS

ABG: arterial blood gas
AG: anion gap
BUN: blood urea nitrogen
CA: carbonic anhydrase enzyme
CHF: congestive heart failure
CNS: central nervous system
COPD: chronic obstructive pulmonary disease
FRC: functional residual capacity
HCl: hydrochloric acid
Hgb: hemoglobin
ICU: intensive care unit
PaO_2: partial pressure of oxygen (mmHg) – arterial
$PaCO_2$: partial pressure of carbon dioxide (mmHg) – arterial
pRBCs: packed red blood cells
RQ: respiratory quotient (VCO_2 / VO_2)
RR: respiratory rate
RTA: renal tubular acidosis
UA: unmeasured anions
UC: unmeasured cations

KEY EQUATIONS

$$AG = UA - UC = Na^+ + K^+ - (Cl^- + HCO_3^-)$$

$$H_2O + CO_2 \overset{CA}{\rightleftarrows} H_2CO_3 \rightleftarrows H^+ + HCO_3^-$$

INTERPRETING THE ARTERIAL BLOOD GAS

pH / $Paco_2$ / Pao_2 / HCO_3 / base deficit
(normal = 7.35–7.45 / 40 / 100 / 24 / 0)

Note: The HCO_3 on an ABG is a *calculated* number. You should use the serum chemistry *measured* value of HCO_3 for a more accurate interpretation of an ABG.

Correct Terminology

▶ Blood pH is normal, *acidemic*, or *alkalemic* (not acidotic or alkalotic).

▶ A patient is acidemic secondary to a process of either *metabolic acidosis* or *respiratory acidosis,* or is alkalemic secondary to a process of *metabolic alkalosis* or *respiratory alkalosis.*

• It is incorrect to say that a patient is *acidotic* or *alkalotic.*

Is the Patient Acidemic or Alkalemic?

▶ pH < 7.35 = acidemia
▶ pH > 7.45 = alkalemia

Is It a Primary Metabolic or Respiratory Process?

See Table 8-1.

TABLE 8-1.
METABOLIC AND RESPIRATORY PROCESSES

Condition	pH	$Paco_2$	HCO_3
Metabolic acidosis	↓	↓	↓
Metabolic alkalosis	↑	↑	↑
Respiratory acidosis	↓	↑	↑
Respiratory alkalosis	↑	↓	↓

Note: A change of 10 mmHg in the $Paco_2$ usually shifts the pH by 0.08 in the opposite direction.

Note: Respiratory compensation is usually a rapid process, whereas metabolic compensation takes time to occur. If the compensation is inappropriate, you should consider a mixed metabolic and respiratory process.

Is the Patient's Compensation Appropriate?

See Table 8-2.

TABLE 8-2.
COMPENSATION

Condition	Metabolic compensation	Respiratory compensation
Metabolic acidosis	None	$PaCO_2$ should decrease 1.0–1.5× decrease in HCO_3^-
Metabolic alkalosis	None	$PaCO_2$ should increase 0.25–1.0× increase in HCO_3^-
Acute respiratory acidosis	HCO_3^- should increase by 1 per 10 increase in $PaCO_2$	None
Chronic respiratory acidosis	HCO_3^- should increase by 4 per 10 increase in $PaCO_2$	None
Acute respiratory alkalosis	HCO_3^- should decrease by 1–3 per 10 decrease in $PaCO_2$	None
Chronic respiratory alkalosis	HCO_3^- should decrease by 2–5 per 10 decrease in $PaCO_2$	None

Base Deficit (or Excess)

▶ *Measured* value on the blood gas.
▶ Use this number to assess the *degree* of *metabolic* acidosis or alkalosis.
  • Deficit (negative number) = acidosis.
  • Excess (positive number) = alkalosis.

Calculating the Anion Gap

$$AG = UA - UC = Na^+ + K^+ - (Cl^- + HCO_3^-)$$

▶ Normal AG = 7–15 (varies per individual laboratory)
- Common UA
  - Proteins (albumin)
  - Sulfate (SO_4^-)
  - Phosphate (PO_4^-)
  - Organic acids
- Common UC
  - Magnesium (Mg^{2+})
  - Calcium (Ca^{2+})
- Increased AG
  - Due to increased UA, decreased UC, or both
    - Examples: lactic acidosis (increased lactate), hypocalcemia
- Decreased AG
  - Due to decreased UA, increased UC, or both
    - Examples: hypoalbuminemia, hypercalcemia, multiple myeloma [which increases the number of positively charged immunoglobulin M (IgM) antibodies]

REVIEW OF THE NEPHRON (THE BASICS)

Proximal Convoluted Tubule

▶ Reabsorbs ~85% of the filtered bicarbonate (HCO_3^-), which is linked to a Na^+/H^+ exchange (sodium reabsorbed and hydrogen secreted)
▶ Reabsorbs chloride (Cl^-) along with Na^+ to maintain electrical neutrality
▶ Reabsorbs 67% of the filtered Na^+ and H_2O

Loop of Henle (Thick Ascending Limb)

▶ Reabsorbs 20% of the filtered Na^+ using a Na^+, K^+, $2Cl^-$ co-transporter
▶ Impermeable to H_2O

Distal Tubule and Collecting Duct

▶ Reabsorbs 12% of the filtered Na^+
▶ Reabsorbs H_2O (antidiuretic hormone mediated)

- Principal cells
  - Na^+ reabsorption and K^+ secretion (aldosterone mediated)
- Intercalated cells
  - K^+ reabsorption and H^+ secretion (aldosterone mediated)

  Note: Remember, extra-renal cells also maintain a K^+/H^+ exchange to maintain homeostasis between intra- and extra-cellular potassium and hydrogen ions.

METABOLIC ACIDOSIS

Normal Anion Gap Acidosis

Hyperchloremic acidosis due to a loss of HCO_3^- or excessive Cl^- intake

Etiology
- Diarrhea
  - Lose bicarbonate in the stool
- Renal tubular acidosis (RTA)
  - Type I (distal RTA)
    - Physiology
      - Defect in the intercalated cells that inhibits adequate H^+ secretion.
      - Urine pH increases.
      - Usually accompanied by hypokalemia.
    - Causes in the ICU
      - Sickle cell disease, chronic active hepatitis, hypercalcemia, renal disease (transplant rejection, obstructive uropathy), drugs (amphotericin B, lithium)
    - Treatment
      - If the patient is severely acidemic (e.g., pH < 7.25), you can administer exogenous bicarbonate.
  - Type II (proximal RTA)
    - Physiology
      - Proximal convoluted tubule cannot adequately reabsorb HCO_3^-.
      - Urine pH increases.
      - Usually accompanied with hypokalemia.
    - Causes in the ICU
      - Drugs (acetazolamide), amyloidosis, myeloma

- ○ Treatment
  - ▪ Shohl's solution (potassium citrate):
    - ➢ Protects against the hypokalemia associated with a proximal RTA.
    - ➢ The citrate is converted to bicarbonate by the liver.
  - ▪ Exogenous bicarbonate administration is *not* recommended.
    - ➢ Can increase the filtered load of HCO_3^- and thus increase the excreted load in the urine, which can potentially worsen the hypokalemia.
- Type IV RTA (hyporenin hypoaldosteronism)
  - ○ Physiology
    - ▪ Decreased action of aldosterone on the collecting duct which thereby cannot adequately secrete H^+.
    - ▪ Associated with hyperkalemia.
  - ○ Causes in the ICU
    - ▪ Chronic renal disease such as diabetic nephropathy, obstructive uropathy, sickle cell disease, Addison's disease (adrenal insufficiency).
  - ○ Treatment
    - ▪ Treat the hyperkalemia.
    - ▪ Administer exogenous mineralocorticoids.
      - ➢ Replaces the deficient aldosterone effect
- ▶ Iatrogenic
  - Drugs
    - ○ Acetazolamide (Diamox) – carbonic anhydrase inhibitor
      - ▪ Decreases the proximal reabsorption of bicarbonate.
  - Excessive chloride administration
    - ○ Excessive administration of 0.9 normal saline (Cl^- 154 mEq/L)
  - Total parenteral nutrition (see Chap. 9)
    - ○ Excessive chloride administration
    - ○ Insufficient bicarbonate administration
- ▶ Ureteral diversion
  - Ureterosigmoidostomy

Increased Anion Gap Acidosis

See Table 8-3.

TABLE 8-3.
INCREASED ANION GAP ACIDOSIS MNEMONIC

Mnemonic	Condition	Unmeasured anion
M	Methanol ingestion	Formic acid
U	Uremia	Sulfates, phosphates
D	Diabetic ketoacidosis	Ketoacids (acetoacetate, β-hydroxybutyrate
P	Paraldehyde ingestion	Acetic acid
I	Isoniazid ingestion, isopropyl alcohol ingestion (severe only)	Lactic acid
L	Lactic acidosis	Lactic acid
E	Ethylene glycol ingestion; ethanol ingestion	Glycolic and oxalic acid; ketoacids
S	Salicylate toxicity (aspirin)	Salicylic acid

OSMOLAR GAP

Usually produced by methanol, ethylene glycol, and isopropyl alcohol ingestion (can also be seen with pseudohyponatremia secondary to hyperlipidemia and hyperproteinemia).

Determining Osmolar Gap

▶ First, calculate the estimated serum osmolality.
  • 2(Na) + glucose / 18 + BUN / 2.8
▶ Next, directly measure the serum osmolality (laboratory measurement).
▶ If the *measured* serum osmolality is greater than the *calculated* osmolality by > 10–15 mOsm/kg and the patient has a high AG acidosis, you must consider ingestion of methanol, ethylene glycol, or isopropyl alcohol as the source of acidosis.

Note: Regarding isopropyl alcohol ingestion, usually only a massive amount causes an increased AG acidosis due to a production of lactic acid secondary to cardiac depression and a hypoperfusion to tissues.

Treatment

▶ Methanol and ethylene glycol
  • Supportive management
    ○ Fluids, pressors, intubation, etc.

- ○ Fomepizole
  - ▪ Blocks the alcohol dehydrogenase enzyme, which then reduces the production of toxic metabolites
- ○ Ethanol drip
  - ▪ Competes for the alcohol dehydrogenase enzyme, which also reduces the production of toxic metabolites
- ○ Hemodialysis
  - ▪ Directly clears the toxins from the blood
► Isopropyl alcohol
- • Supportive management
  - ○ Fluids, pressors, intubation, etc.
- • Hemodialysis
  - ○ Directly clears isopropyl alcohol from the blood

Note: Bicarbonate therapy for AG acidemia should be reserved for a pH ≤ 7.20–7.25. Also, you must ensure that the patient has adequate ventilation to remove the carbon dioxide produced by the buffering effect of HCO_3^-. However, if the acidemia is a direct result of bicarbonate *losses* (e.g., diarrhea, pancreatic fistula), then it should be repleted.

$$H_2O + CO_2 \rightleftarrows H_2CO_3 \rightleftarrows H^+ + HCO_3^-$$

Clinical Correlation

A 36-year-old woman with no significant medical history is brought to the emergency room by her friend after she is found to be extremely lethargic and minimally responsive while sitting alone in her car. Her vital signs on arrival are the following: temperature: 37°C (98.6°F), BP 105/70, HR 105, RR 28, SaO_2 97%. She is now unresponsive; thus, you quickly intubate her, obtain IV access, and start aggressive fluid resuscitation. Her laboratory values return as those shown in Table 8-4.

TABLE 8-4.
LABORATORY VALUES

White blood cells	Hgb	Hematocrit	Platelets
7.6	12.3	36.8	326

Na	K	Cl	HCO_3	BUN	Creatinine	Glucose
136	4.0	106	12	9	0.5	105

ABG on room air prior to intubation: 7.20 / 30 / 96 / 14 / –9 / 97%
You quickly calculate her AG to be 22 and determine that she has
an increased AG metabolic acidosis. You rule out uremia (due to
normal renal function) and diabetic ketoacidosis (due to a normal
glucose level) as possible etiologies. A toxicology screen (including
ethanol and salicylates) is sent, which also is negative for any sub-
stance use. A lactate level also returns normal.

The patient's sister arrives at the ICU in a panic demanding to
know how her sister is doing. While explaining the situation to her,
you learn that the patient is currently going through a terrible
divorce and her only child died from lymphoma two months earlier. Suddenly you realize that this is likely a suicide attempt; since
she was found in her car, she likely ingested ethylene glycol (anti-
freeze). You immediately calculate her estimated serum osmolality
to be 281 mOsm/kg and find that her measured serum osmolality
is 307 mOsm/kg, giving her an osmolar gap of 26. You administer
fomepizole and consult the renal team for emergent dialysis. Over
the next three days, the patient dramatically improves and awakens
neurologically intact.

METABOLIC ALKALOSIS

Etiology

▶ Dehydration
  • Contraction alkalosis
▶ Gastrointestinal HCl acid loss
  • Vomiting
  • Nasogastric tube drainage
▶ Chloride losses
  • Compensatory increase in HCO_3^- reabsorption to maintain
    electrical neutrality
▶ Shift of extracellular H^+ into cells
  • Occurs due to extracellular hypokalemia (remember, cells
    maintain a K^+/H^+ exchange)
  • Often secondary to diuretic therapy
▶ Renal H^+ secretion
  • Hypokalemia
  • Diuretics [e.g., furosemide (Lasix)]

- Mineralocorticoid excess (hyperaldosteronism)
  - Aldosterone secreting adrenal tumor (Conn syndrome)
  - A relative increase in aldosterone postoperatively (normal stress response) is further compounded by the administration of a diuretic (e.g., Lasix), which increases the delivery of Na^+ to the distal nephron and leads to an increase in aldosterone-mediated renal H^+ secretion.
- ► Excessive serum HCO_3^-
  - Iatrogenic administration
  - Blood transfusions
    - pRBCs are stored with citrate to prevent clotting.
      - Citrate binds calcium, which is needed for the coagulation cascade.
      - Citrate is then transfused to the patient along with the pRBCs and is then converted to bicarbonate by the liver.

Effects of Alkalemia

- ► Shifts oxygen–Hgb disassociation curve to the left (see Chap. 3).
  - This shift decreases oxygen delivery to peripheral tissues.
- ► Decreases the respiratory drive.
  - Can cause short shallow breaths.
  - Can lead to the FRC being less than closing volume which can cause atelectasis (see Chap. 4).
- ► Enzymes do not function well at a high pH.
- ► Certain medications (e.g., pressors) do not function well at a high pH.

Treatment

- ► Replete K and Cl
  - Be aware of the following conditions that are *unresponsive* to chloride repletion:
    - Hyperaldosteronism
    - Cushing's syndrome
    - Exogenous steroids (including excessive licorice ingestion, which has mineralocorticoid agonist activity)
    - Bartter's syndrome

▶ Administer acetazolamide (Diamox)
  • Carbonic anhydrase inhibitor
  • Increases renal HCO_3^- excretion by inhibiting PCT reabsorption
▶ Administer HCl
  • Reserve this maneuver for severe alkalemia (pH $\geq$ 7.55)
  • Dosing (given IV via a central venous catheter):
    ○ Calculate H^+ ion deficit (mEq) = 0.3 * wt (kg) *
       [measured HCO_3^- – desired HCO_3^- (mEq/L)]
    ○ Use a 0.1 N HCl solution, which contains 100 mEq/L
    ○ Maximum infusion rate = 100 mEq/12 hours
    ○ Usually replace two-thirds of deficit to avoid excessive
       proton administration

RESPIRATORY ACIDOSIS

Etiology

▶ Lung problem
  • Increased dead space (e.g., COPD, asthma)
    ○ Exacerbated by ↑ carbon dioxide production
      ▪ Fever
      ▪ Infection
      ▪ Pregnancy
      ▪ Excessive carbohydrate intake
        ➢ Overfeeding – ↑ RQ (see Chap. 9)
      ▪ Seizures
▶ Pleural disease
  • Effusions
  • Pneumothorax
  • Constrictive pleuritis
▶ CNS depression
  • Cortical
    ○ Sedation (medications, drugs, ethanol)
    ○ Cerebral vascular accident
    ○ Tumor
    ○ Trauma
    ○ Infection
  • Brainstem
    ○ Herniation
    ○ Trauma

▶ Nerve problem
  • Polio
  • Transverse myelitis
  • Amyotrophic lateral sclerosis
  • Guillain-Barré syndrome
  • High cervical spinal cord injury
▶ Neuromuscular junction problem
  • Myasthenia gravis
▶ Chest wall restriction
  • Kyphoscoliosis, flail chest, chest wall edema secondary to massive fluid resuscitation
▶ Muscle disease
  • Muscular dystrophies, hypophosphatemia, fatigue
▶ Decreased respiratory effort secondary to incisional pain
  • Most severe with thoracotomy, subcostal, and upper abdominal incisions

Treatment

▶ Correct the underlying pathology.
▶ Use mechanical ventilation if necessary.

RESPIRATORY ALKALOSIS

Etiology

Usually secondary to a rapid respiratory rate
▶ Lung problem
  • Pneumonia
  • Asthma exacerbation (early in the clinical course)
  • CHF (early in the clinical course)
  • Pulmonary embolism
▶ CNS
  • Infection (meningitis, encephalitis)
  • Severe head trauma
  • Cerebral vascular accident
  • Tumor
▶ Metabolic disorders
  • Sepsis
  • Hyperthyroidism
  • Liver failure

- • Severe anemia
- • High altitude
- • Hypoxemia
- • Fever
▶ Drugs
  - • Salicylates
  - • Paraldehyde
▶ Pregnancy
▶ Iatrogenic
  - • Mechanical over-ventilation
▶ Anxiety
  - • Diagnosis of exclusion

Treatment

▶ Correct the underlying pathology.
▶ Use mechanical ventilation if necessary.
▶ Sedation/anxiolytics.

CHAPTER 9

NUTRITION

ABBREVIATIONS

BMR: basal metabolic rate
CNS: central nervous system
DVT: deep venous thrombosis
ICU: intensive care unit
RQ: respiratory quotient (V_{CO_2} / V_{O_2})
TPN: total parenteral nutrition
UUN: urinary urea nitrogen
V_{CO_2}: production of carbon dioxide (ml CO_2/min)
V_{O_2}: consumption of oxygen (ml O_2/min)

ENTERAL NUTRITION

Advantages

▶ Most physiologic method for providing nutrition.
▶ Less costly than TPN.
▶ Maintains the integrity of bowel mucosa.
▶ The benefit of trophic feeds (i.e., tube feeding at 10 cc/hr) is controversial.
  • The theoretical benefit of a reduction in the risk of bacterial translocation is still debated.
  • It provides a method for delivering glutamine, which is believed to be essential for bowel mucosa integrity.
  • Regardless of whether it is beneficial, trophic feeding is *not harmful* if the patient can tolerate it.
▶ Administering enteral nutrition *early* in a patient's clinical course has been shown to significantly decrease the acute phase response to injury [systemic inflammatory response syndrome (SIRS)] compared to TPN.
  • Decreases levels of C-reactive protein and oxidant stress.
  • Reduces the incidence of septic complications.
  • Decreases the incidence of multiple organ dysfunction syndrome (MODS).

Contraindications

- Clinical shock
- Complete bowel obstruction
- Intestinal ischemia
- Severe paralytic ileus
- *High output* (> 500 cc/day) enterocutaneous fistula (This is a relative contraindication and is practitioner dependent.)

Methods of Feeding

Gastric
- ► Nasogastric tube
  - Large-caliber tube
  - Has a sump port
    - ○ Enables the tube to be placed to wall suction without injuring or directly applying suction to the gastric mucosa
    - ○ Enables the monitoring of a *gastric residual volume*
- ► Gastrostomy tube
  - Does not have a sump port
    - ○ Cannot be placed to wall suction
    - ○ Collection bag can be placed to gravity to check a residual volume
- ► Small-caliber feeding tube (Dobhoff tube)
  - Intended to be placed in the duodenum, but it can also be placed in the stomach
  - Does not have a sump port
    - ○ Cannot be placed to wall suction
    - ○ Residual volumes cannot be checked

Note: Using the "gastric residual volume" to titrate the rate of administering tube feeds is poorly standardized. There is no clear correlation between a certain residual volume and the incidence of pulmonary aspiration, but a residual volume of 200–250 cc is often used clinically.

Duodenal (Post-Pyloric)
- ► Nasoduodenal tube (also called a Dobhoff tube)
  - Small-caliber tube
    - ○ Has a weighted end that facilitates passage past the pylorus

- Allows enteral feeding in patients with a poorly functioning stomach
- Does not have a sump port
  - Cannot be placed to wall suction
  - Residual volumes cannot be checked

Jejunal
► Nasojejunal tube
  - Small-caliber tube
  - Allows enteral feeding in patients with a poorly functioning stomach
  - Does not have a sump port
    - Cannot be placed to wall suction
    - Residual volumes cannot be checked
► Jejunostomy tube
  - Does not have a sump port
    - Cannot be placed to wall suction
    - Residual volumes cannot be checked
► Gastrojejunostomy tube
  - Double-lumen tube that allows gastric gravity drainage and jejunal feeding simultaneously.
  - The proximal port is left in the stomach for gravity drainage and the distal tip is placed in the jejunum for feeding.
  - Does not have a sump port.
    - The proximal gastric port cannot be placed to wall suction.

Note: You do not need to check "residual volumes" when feeding the patient distal to the stomach. There is no anatomic reservoir in the small bowel from which to measure a residual volume. Also, the feeding tubes designed for distal feeding usually do not have a sump port, and thus you cannot check a residual volume. The rate of infusion should be titrated to clinical signs such as diarrhea and abdominal distention.

Methods of Placing Feeding Tubes

Bedside
► Used for nasogastric, nasoduodenal, and nasojejunal feeding tubes.

▶ Advantages
  • No need to transport the patient
  • Rapid insertion
▶ Disadvantages
  • Relatively blind procedure.
  • When distal feeding is desired, it is difficult to guide the tube into the duodenum and jejunum because it relies on gut peristalsis. Radiographic assistance is often required to position the tube properly into either the duodenum or jejunum.

Note: After placing a feeding tube at the bedside, you should **always** confirm proper placement of the tube with an x-ray **before** starting feeds to avoid the dangerous situation of infusing feeds directly into the lungs or esophagus, where they may be aspirated.

Endoscopic

▶ Used for percutaneous gastrostomy tubes, nasojejunal tubes, and nasogastrojejunal double-lumen tubes
▶ Advantages
  • Can be performed at the bedside and does not require any patient transport.
  • The feeding tubes are placed with direct endoscopic guidance.
▶ Disadvantages
  • Minimally invasive procedure.
  • There is a small but real risk of bowel perforation secondary to traumatic endoscope insertion.

Radiographic

▶ Used for gastrostomy tubes, nasoduodenal and nasojejunal tubes, and percutaneous gastrojejunostomy double-lumen tubes
▶ Advantages
  • Able to confirm proper position of the feeding tube during placement.
▶ Disadvantages
  • It usually requires transporting the patient to the radiology suite.
  • The tube is not placed under direct vision.
  • There is a small but real risk of bowel perforation, usually from a traumatic guidewire insertion.

Surgical
▶ Used for gastrostomy tubes, jejunostomy tubes, and gastrojejunostomy double-lumen tubes.
▶ Advantages
  • The feeding tubes are placed under direct vision.
▶ Disadvantages
  • Requires transporting the patient to the operating room.
  • Usually requires administering general anesthesia to the patient; however, the procedure can sometimes be performed using local anesthesia.

Tube Feeding Considerations

Volume
▶ You usually start with a low rate of infusion and slowly increase to goal.
▶ The goal rate is determined by the total caloric needs of the patient and the type of formula being fed.
▶ The goal rate can be *estimated* by infusing the same amount per hour as the patient's weight in kilograms.
  • Example: When using a 1 kcal/cc formula, the goal rate of a 60-kg patient can be estimated at 60 cc/hr. This is halved when using a concentrated formula that contains 2 kcal/cc.

Osmolarity
▶ You can use half-, three-fourths-, or full-strength feedings.
  • You should consider the location of feeding when deciding upon osmolarity.
    ○ Stomach – Full strength feeds are usually tolerated
    ○ Jejunum – Consider decreasing the osmolarity of the feeds in order to avoid diarrhea
  • You can also start with a low osmolarity and slowly increase it to full strength feeds if the patient tolerates it.
  • The use of initial full strength jejunal feeding in patients with hypotension or compromised bowel can be associated with bowel infarction.

Note: Tube feeding–induced diarrhea can be secondary to either excessive volumes or excessive osmolarity.

Types of Formulas
▶ Standard
  • 1 kcal/cc
  • Low cost
▶ Elemental
  • 1 kcal/cc
  • Costly
  • Low protein, high carbohydrate
  • High osmolarity
▶ Semi-elemental
  • 1 kcal/cc
  • More costly
  • High protein
▶ Volume restricted
  • 2 kcal/cc
  • Low cost
▶ Renal formula (for patients with renal failure)
  • 2 kcal/cc (enables you to deliver adequate nutrition with low volumes)
  • Low potassium
  • Low protein
  • Low cost
▶ Critical care formulas
  • 1 kcal/cc
  • Contain immune-enhancing substances
    ○ Examples: fish oils, RNA, and arginine
  • High cost

Note: The choice of formula should be based on each patient's specific needs and clinical situation.

Risk of Pulmonary Aspiration

▶ There is no clear difference in the incidence of pulmonary aspiration between gastric and post-pyloric (i.e., duodenal) feeding.
▶ Jejunal feeding (i.e., post ligament of Treitz) theoretically offers a lower risk of pulmonary aspiration; however, large randomized clinical trials still need to be performed.
▶ Gastric residual volumes are poorly standardized and do not correlate well with incidence of pulmonary aspiration.

► Pulmonary aspiration can also occur *antegrade* from oropharyngeal secretions as well as retrograde from the stomach.
► Methods of minimizing the risk of pulmonary aspiration and subsequent aspiration pneumonia:
  • Administer antiseptics to achieve oral decontamination, which can reduce the incidence of aspiration pneumonia.
  • Avoid placing the patient in the supine position.
  • Keep the head of bed above 30–45 degrees.
  • When using nasally inserted feeding tubes, use small-caliber tubes because they theoretically do not "stent open" the lower esophageal sphincter as much as a large-caliber tube does. This can theoretically reduce the incidence of aspiration.
  • Ensure proper nursing education in methods to prevent pulmonary aspiration.

PARENTERAL NUTRITION

Indications
► The patient cannot tolerate enteral nutrition.
  • You can use TPN to supplement enteral nutrition to deliver a patient's goal calories.
► Severely malnourished patients scheduled to undergo major abdominal surgery should receive appropriate nutrition for 5–7 days preoperatively. If you cannot use enteral nutrition in this situation, then use TPN.
► Administer TPN if you are unable to deliver enteral nutrition after 7 days postoperatively.
  • You should use it after 48 hours for critically ill patients.

How to Write Parenteral Nutrition

Calculate the Patient's Goal Calories
► Normal conditions: 25 kcal/kg/day
► Stressed patient (e.g., critically ill): 30–35 kcal/kg/day

Protein
► Contains 4 kcal/g
► Normal conditions: 0.8–1.0 g/kg/day

▶ Stressed patient: 1.5–2.0 g/kg/day
▶ You should reduce the protein content for patients with renal failure.

Carbohydrates

▶ Contains 3.4 kcal/g
▶ Usual dose range: 3–5 g/kg/day
  • You can deliver the balance of [goal calories – protein calories] as carbohydrates.
  • You can also deliver the balance of [goal calories – (protein + fat calories)] as carbohydrates.
▶ You should usually start with a low rate of glucose infusion and titrate to goal calories.
  • You must monitor and control serum glucose levels tightly (goal is to maintain < 120 mg/dl).
  • Use insulin aggressively to control hyperglycemia.
    ○ Reduces the risk of infection.
▶ Excessive carbohydrate loading can increase the RQ (V_{CO_2} / V_{O_2}) and predispose the patient to respiratory dysfunction from excessive carbon dioxide production.

Fats

▶ Contains 9 kcal/g
▶ Usual dose range: 1.0–1.5 g/kg/day
▶ Usually limited to 30% of a patient's total calories.
▶ You should monitor the serum triglyceride level (must be < 400 mg/dl).
▶ You can administer fats every day or every other day (practitioner dependent).
  • Administered as a 3:1 solution (all components mixed in one bag) or separately over 12 hours.
  • Potential complications of excessive fat administration:
    ○ Can overload the reticuloendothelial system.
    ○ Can increase the risk of infection.
  • Potential benefits:
    ○ Decreases de novo lipogenesis.
    ○ Allows you to decrease the glucose load for diabetics while still providing goal calories.
    ○ Prevents essential fatty acid deficiency (oleic and linoleic fatty acids).

- ○ Decreases carbon dioxide production (RQ of fat = 0.7).
- ○ Decreases the osmolarity of the 3:1 solution.
  - ▪ Reduces the risk of phlebitis.
- ○ Decreases the volume required to deliver goal calories.

Electrolytes
See Table 9-1.

TABLE 9-1.
ELECTROLYTES

Electrolyte	Usual adult daily IV dose	Recommended daily allowance adult PO dose
Sodium	100–150 mEq	22 mEq
Potassium	60–120 mEq	40–50 mEq
Chloride	100–150 mEq	22 mEq
Calcium	9–22 mEq	20–30 mEq
Phosphorus	15–30 mEq	26–39 mEq
Magnesium	8–24 mEq	11.5–14.4 mEq

Note: You must adjust the electrolyte composition of TPN for each patient's electrolyte profile.

Additives in Parenteral Nutrition
- ▶ Heparin
  - • 6000–12,000 units/day.
  - • Can prevent catheter-related venous thrombosis.
  - • Also used for DVT prophylaxis.
  - • Some practitioners prefer to administer heparin separately and not add it to the TPN bag. This enables you to adjust the heparin dose without having to waste the entire bag of TPN for that day.
- ▶ Histamine-2 blockers
  - • Used for stress ulcer prophylaxis.
- ▶ Insulin
  - • Used for controlling serum glucose levels.
- ▶ Promotility agents [metoclopramide (Reglan)]
  - • Can aid in shifting the patient's nutrition to enteral feeding.
- ▶ Zinc
  - • This mineral promotes wound healing.

▶ Vitamin K
  • Usually added once a week to the solution (10 mg/wk) to maintain an adequate level of vitamin K–dependent coagulation factors (II, VII, IX, X, protein C, protein S) and a functioning coagulation cascade. Be careful in patients on warfarin (Coumadin) therapy.

Clinical Correlation

A 67-year-old man weighing 55 kg and with a history of alcohol abuse is admitted with necrotizing pancreatitis. He tells you that he does not have a home and has not had a decent meal in 3 weeks. On examination, he is hypotensive and tachycardic, and his abdomen is distended with minimal bowel sounds. He is admitted to the ICU, central IV access is obtained, and appropriate management is started. Due to his malnourished state, you decide to start TPN. Knowing that he is in a severely catabolic state from his illness, you begin calculating his calorie requirements accordingly.

$$\text{Goal kcal} = 35 \text{ kcal/kg/day} * 55 \text{ kg}$$
$$= 1925 \text{ kcal/day}$$
$$\text{Protein requirement} = 2 \text{ g/kg/day} * 55 \text{ kg}$$
$$= 110 \text{ g/day}$$
$$\text{kcal from protein} = 110 \text{ g} * 4 \text{ kcal/g}$$
$$= 440 \text{ kcal}$$
$$\text{Goal kcal} - \text{protein kcal} = 1925 \text{ kcal} - 440 \text{ kcal}$$
$$= 1485 \text{ kcal}$$

You check his triglyceride level to rule it out as a cause for his pancreatitis, and it returns normal. So, you decide to administer fats in his TPN as 30% of his goal calories.

$$\text{kcal from fat} = \text{goal kcal} * 0.30$$
$$= 1925 \text{ kcal} * 0.30$$
$$= 576 \text{ kcal}$$
$$\text{Grams of fat} = \text{fat kcal} / 9 \text{ kcal/g}$$
$$= 576 \text{ kcal} / 9 \text{ kcal/g}$$
$$= 64 \text{ g}$$

Next, you calculate his carbohydrate requirement in order to deliver his goal calories.

$$\text{Carbohydrate kcal} = \text{goal kcal} - (\text{protein} + \text{fat kcal})$$

$$= 1925 \text{ kcal} - (440 + 576 \text{ kcal})$$

$$= 909 \text{ kcal}$$

$$\text{Grams of carbohydrate} = \text{carbohydrate kcal} / 3.4 \text{ kcal/g}$$

$$= 909 \text{ kcal} / 3.4 \text{ kcal/g}$$

$$= 267 \text{ g}$$

You start off with a carbohydrate load of 150 g/day to monitor and control his serum glucose levels. Over the next 2 days, you increase the carbohydrates in the TPN to deliver his goal calories and find that he requires 45 units of insulin/day to control his serum glucose levels. His abdominal distention is improved and he is now passing flatus per rectum. However, his mid-epigastrium remains tender. You want to start administering enteral nutrition, so you ask your radiology colleagues to place a nasojejunal feeding tube under fluoroscopic guidance. This allows you to administer enteral feeds without stimulating pancreatic enzyme secretions because the tip of the feeding tube is distal to the ligament of Treitz. You begin half-strength Impact, a critical care formula, at 10 cc/hr.

Over the next 2 days, the patient tolerates the enteral feeds well, and you are able to wean the TPN and increase his tube feeds to full strength at 55 cc/hr, thus delivering his goal calories enterally. TPN is discontinued, and he is maintained on complete enteral nutrition. Over the next 5 days, his clinical status improves and he is started on enteral nutrition per mouth. He tolerates this well and is slowly advanced to a regular diet while his tube feeds are weaned and finally discontinued.

Potential Complications of Administering Total Parenteral Nutrition

Hyperglycemia
▶ Increases the risk of infection
▶ Increases carbon dioxide production
▶ Increases de novo hepatic lipogenesis
▶ Induces osmotic diuresis

► Treatment
  • Administer aggressive insulin therapy
    ○ Goal glucose is ≤ 120 mg/dl
  • Reduce the carbohydrate load in the TPN if necessary

Hypertriglyceridemia
► Can overload the reticuloendothelial system
► Potential risk of pancreatitis
► Potential CNS toxicity
► Treatment
  • Remove fats from the TPN

Electrolyte Abnormalities
► Potential CNS toxicity
► Treatment
  • Adjust electrolytes appropriately in the TPN

Note: You must monitor for refeeding syndrome in patients with severe malnutrition who are starting TPN. This syndrome is characterized by severe electrolyte abnormalities, such as hypophosphatemia, hypokalemia, hypomagnesemia, and fluid retention. Any electrolyte abnormalities must be corrected before administering high-glucose solutions.

Central Line Related
► Infection
  • You must use sterile technique for line insertion and apply proper site care
► Air embolism
► Pneumothorax during line placement

Gut Changes
► There is a potential for intestinal mucosal atrophy because of disuse.
  • You should convert to enteral nutrition as soon as the patient can tolerate it.
► There is also a potential for *acalculous* cholecystitis secondary to biliary stasis.
  • Treat in the same manner as calculous cholecystitis.

ASSESSING NUTRITIONAL STATUS

Nitrogen Balance

▶ Nitrogen balance =
nitrogen input – (UUN + 4)

> Nitrogen input = grams of protein intake / 6.25
> UUN = grams in 24-hour urine collection
> (1 g UUN = 6.25 g protein)

- If nitrogen balance is 0 to –5 g/day
  ○ Patient is in moderate stress.
- If nitrogen balance is more than –5 g/day
  ○ Patient is in severe stress.

Harris Benedict Formula

▶ Estimates BMR using height, weight, gender, and age
- Female
  ○ BMR (calories) = 655 + (9.6 * weight in kg) + (1.8 * height in cm) – (4.7 * age in years)
- Male
  ○ BMR (calories) = 66 + (13.7 * weight in kg) + (5 * height in cm) – (6.8 * age in years)

Metabolic Cart/Indirect Calorimetry

▶ Measures RQ (V_{CO_2} / V_{O_2}).
▶ Mixed fuel intake RQ = 0.82.
▶ RQ > 1 implies overfeeding.
▶ This technique measures V_{O_2} to estimate energy expenditure.

> RQ is affected by dietary intake
> Fat: RQ = 0.7
> Protein: RQ = 0.8
> Carbohydrate: RQ = 1.0

- Burning 1 calorie (kcal) requires 208.06 ml of oxygen.
- A patient's energy expenditure can be used to adjust the nutritional support accordingly.

CHAPTER 10

PROPHYLAXIS AGAINST DEEP VENOUS THROMBOSIS AND STRESS ULCERATION

ABBREVIATIONS

COPD: chronic obstructive pulmonary disease
DVT: deep venous thrombosis
HIT: heparin-induced thrombocytopenia
INR: international normalized ratio
PA: pulmonary artery

DEEP VENOUS THROMBOSIS PROPHYLAXIS

Risk Factors

- ► Increased age
- ► African American > white > Latino > Asian
- ► Surgical procedures
  - High risk
    - ○ Orthopedic surgery involving a hip repair
    - ○ Neurosurgery
    - ○ Major vascular procedures, major bowel surgery, major pelvic surgery, obesity surgery
    - ○ Long operations
  - Low risk
    - ○ Laparoscopic cholecystectomy and appendectomy
    - ○ Neck surgery (thyroid, parathyroid)
    - ○ Inguinal hernia repair
    - ○ Short operations
- ► History of prior DVT
- ► Thrombophilic disorder

- Factor V Leiden (most common)
- Antiphospholipid antibody
  - Lupus anticoagulant
  - Anticardiolipin antibody
- Antithrombin III deficiency
- Protein C deficiency
- Protein S deficiency
- Hyperhomocysteinemia (accompanied by homocysteinuria)
▶ Malignancy
▶ Obesity
▶ Comorbidities
  - Congestive heart failure
  - COPD
▶ Immobilization

Treatment Options

Nonpharmacologic
▶ Early ambulation
▶ Elastic stockings
▶ Intermittent pneumatic compression devices
  - Should not be used as the only agent in high-risk patients unless anticoagulation is contraindicated
  - Often used in conjunction with pharmacologic modalities because of a presumed "additive" benefit
  - May have reduced efficacy in obese patients

Pharmacologic
▶ Heparin
  - Mechanism of action
    - Binds to antithrombin and catalyzes the inactivation of several activated coagulation factors, including Xa and IIa (thrombin)
  - Recommended doses
    - Moderate risk: 5000 IU SC q 8–12 hours
    - High risk: 5000 IU SC q 6–8 hours
  - Potential complications
    - There is a slightly higher risk of bleeding compared to using low-molecular-weight heparin.

- ○ Heparin-induced thrombocytopenia (HIT)
  - ▪ HIT-I
    - ➢ Occurs in 10–20% of patients.
    - ➢ Usually causes an approximately 20–50% reduction in platelet levels.
    - ➢ Usually is self-limited, and no specific treatment is required.
    - ➢ Heparin should be stopped until HIT-II (see below) is definitively excluded.
  - ▪ HIT-II
    - ➢ Occurs in < 1–3% of patients.
    - ➢ Usually causes a marked reduction in platelet levels secondary to immune-mediated platelet-rich diffuse arterial thrombosis.
    - ➢ Leads to severe bleeding and clotting complications.
    - ➢ Treatment is to discontinue **all** heparin and heparin-containing products (e.g., heparin-coated PA line).
    - ➢ Do **not** transfuse platelets because HIT-II is a consumptive coagulopathy and transfusing platelets can propel the diffuse thrombosis.
    - ➢ You can substitute heparin with a direct thrombin inhibitor (e.g., hirudin).
- ▶ Low-molecular-weight heparin
  - • Mechanism of action
    - ○ Catalyzes inactivation of factor Xa
  - • Recommended doses
    - ○ Enoxaparin (Lovenox)
      - ▪ 0.5 mg/kg SC q 12 hours
      - ▪ 30 mg SC q 12 hours
      - ▪ 40 mg SC q 24 hours
    - ○ Dalteparin (Fragmin)
      - ▪ Moderate risk: 2500 IU SC q 24 hours
      - ▪ High risk: 5000 IU SC q 24 hours
- ▶ Warfarin (Coumadin)
  - • This is reserved for very high-risk patients, such as those undergoing hip surgery
  - • Recommended INR range: 2.0–2.5

STRESS ULCER PROPHYLAXIS

Pathogenesis

▶ An inadequate blood flow leads to breakdown of the layer of mucus protecting the gastric mucosa.
▶ The underlying mucosa is then eroded by gastric acidity.
  • This is not usually due to increased gastric acid secretion.
  • One exception is in patients with severe head injury, in which acid hypersecretion is a common finding.
▶ These are usually superficial ulcers.
  • They rarely progress to perforation.
  • The major morbidity is from bleeding.

Treatment Options

Gastric Feeding
▶ Ideal method of prophylaxis if gastric motility is intact.
▶ Effective for preventing stress ulcer bleeding.
▶ You must consider each patient's potential risk for aspiration.

Sucralfate (Carafate)
▶ Coats the stomach and protects the mucosa.
▶ Does not change the acidic pH environment of the stomach.
  • The acidity helps to maintain a sterile environment in the stomach.
▶ Ideal if gastric motility is impaired, but not completely absent, because it increases the contact time of sucralfate with the gastric mucosa.

Histamine-2 Blocker
▶ Reduces acid secretion.
  • Increases the pH and potentially allows for bacterial contamination.
  • Theoretically, if the patient aspirates, there can be an increased risk of aspiration pneumonia, as opposed to an aspiration-induced chemical pneumonitis. However, this has not been substantiated in large series.
▶ Preferred over sucralfate when gastric motility is severely compromised.

Proton Pump Inhibitor

► *Markedly* reduces acid secretion by blocking the final common pathway necessary for acid secretion.
  • Potentially allows for bacterial contamination.
  • Potentially increases the risk of aspiration pneumonia vs. aspiration pneumonitis.
► Should be used in patients experiencing gastric stress ulcer bleeding complications or in those who are already taking this medication on an outpatient basis.
► Consider using these agents or histamine-2 blockers for patients with severe head injury, regardless of administration of tube feedings.

MANAGEMENT

Chapters 11–20 address *specific* management issues for the most common disease processes encountered in the intensive care unit. However, every patient in the intensive care unit should be approached in a system-by-system manner:

- Neurologic/pain control
- Cardiovascular
- Pulmonary
- Gastrointestinal
- Renal
- Infectious disease
- Hematologic
- Endocrine
- Fluids and electrolytes
- Nutrition
- Prophylaxis
- Disposition/code status/consideration of organ donation

CHAPTER 11

ACUTE MYOCARDIAL INFARCTION

ABBREVIATIONS

aVF: augmented voltage unipolar left foot lead
aVL: augmented voltage unipolar left arm lead
MI: myocardial infarction
PA: pulmonary artery
PTT: partial thromboplastin time
SaO_2: arterial oxygen saturation

DEFINITION

▶ Necrosis or death of myocardial cells
  • Results from a mismatch of oxygen delivery and oxygen demand
  • Categories
    ○ Transmural infarct
      ▪ Ischemic necrosis of full thickness muscle
    ○ Non-transmural infarct
      ▪ Does not extend full thickness – usually involves the endocardium because it is the area most distant from the blood supply

PATHOPHYSIOLOGY

Risk Factors for Myocardial Infarction

▶ Hypertension
▶ Diabetes mellitus
▶ High blood cholesterol
▶ Tobacco use

▶ Male gender
- Gender difference narrows after women undergo menopause.
▶ Family history of coronary artery disease

Usual Order of Events That Cause Myocardial Infarction

▶ Development of atherosclerotic plaque over years to decades
- Composition of the plaque
  ◦ Fibromuscular cap
  ◦ Underlying lipid-rich core
▶ Disruption of the vessel endothelium
- Can be secondary to collagenase and protease activity
- Can be secondary to hemodynamic forces against the arterial wall
▶ Rupture of the fibromuscular cap
▶ Formation of a thrombus via platelet-mediated activation of the coagulation cascade
- Degree of ischemia is related to the size of the thrombus.

Three Factors That Determine Severity of Myocardial Infarction

▶ Level of occlusion in the coronary artery
- Generally, the more proximal the occlusion, the greater the risk of extensive myocardial necrosis.
▶ Length of time of occlusion
- Myocardial death generally begins in the endocardium.
  ◦ Most distal to the blood supply
- Spreads to myocardium, and eventually to the epicardium.
- Six to 8 hours of ischemia usually lead to myocardial cell death.
- If ischemia time continues, the damaged area can spread laterally to watershed regions.
▶ Presence or absence of collateral circulation
- Presence of collateral circulation reduces infarct size.

SYMPTOMS AND SIGNS

Symptoms

▶ Can be asymptomatic
- Does not mean less myocardial damage

- • Usually occurs in patients with diabetes due to the development of neuropathy
- ▶ Chest pain
  - • Pressure sensation
  - • Feeling of tight squeeze in chest
- ▶ Radiation of chest pain to
  - • Shoulder
  - • Arm
  - • Back
  - • Jaw / teeth
- ▶ Epigastric discomfort
  - • Nausea
  - • Vomiting

Signs

- ▶ Dyspnea
- ▶ Diaphoresis
- ▶ Syncope or near-syncope without other cause
- ▶ Mental status change without other cause
- ▶ Hypotension
  - • Can also be hypertensive or normotensive
- ▶ Tachycardia
  - • Can also be bradycardiac or have a normal heart rate
- ▶ Hypoxia

DIAGNOSIS

- ▶ History and physical examination
- ▶ Electrocardiogram
  - • T-wave inversion
  - • ST-segment depression
  - • ST-segment elevation
    - ◦ Does not distinguish a transmural from a non-transmural infarct
    - ◦ Usually associated with higher early morbidity and mortality
  - • Q waves
    - ◦ Do not distinguish a transmural from a non-transmural infarct
    - ◦ Usually associated with higher early morbidity and mortality

- Dysrhythmias
- Corresponding segments of the left ventricle
  - Lateral wall: I, aVL, V_6
  - Inferior wall: II, III, aVF
  - Anterior wall/septum: V_1–V_5
▶ Blood tests (Table 11-1)
▶ Echocardiography
- Demonstrates areas of wall motion abnormalities
  - Does not differentiate between acute or previous MI
  - Limited role in diagnosis of acute MI

TABLE 11-1.
BLOOD TESTS IN MYOCARDIAL INFARCTION

Enzyme	Normal range
Total CPK	30–200 U/L
CPK, MB fraction	0.0–8.8 ng/ml
CPK, MB fraction percent of total CPK	0–4%
Troponin I	0.0–0.4 ng/ml

CPK, creatinine phosphokinase.
Note: These values may differ for individual laboratories.

MANAGEMENT

Airway

▶ Ensure a stable airway.
- Consider mechanical ventilation if necessary (see Chap. 4).

Oxygenation

▶ Administer supplemental oxygen.
▶ Consider mechanical ventilation if necessary (see Chap. 4).
▶ Maintain $SaO_2 \geq 90\%$.

Aspirin

▶ Administer immediately.
- Irreversible inhibitor of platelet adhesion and cohesion.
▶ Dose: 160–325 mg PO/NG QD.
▶ Proven reduction in mortality.

Other Antiplatelet Agents

Glycoprotein Ia Antagonists
▶ Not shown to be superior to aspirin
▶ Useful for patients with a true allergy to aspirin
▶ Dose
  • Clopidogrel (Plavix): 75 mg PO/NG QD
  • Ticlopidine (Ticlid): 250 mg PO/NG BID
  • Dipyridamole (Persantine): 75–100 mg PO/NG QID

Glycoprotein IIb/IIIa Antagonists
▶ Potent inhibitors of platelet aggregation
▶ Shown to reduce mortality
▶ Dose
  • Eptifibatide (Integrilin)
    ○ Loading dose: 180 μg/kg IV
    ○ Infusion: 2 μg/kg/min * 72 hours
  • Tirofiban (Aggrastat)
    ○ Start 0.4 μg/kg/min * 30 minutes
    ○ Then 0.1 μg/kg/min * 48–108 hours
  • Abciximab (ReoPro)
    ○ Loading dose: 0.25 mg/kg IV
    ○ Infusion: 0.125 μg/kg/min IV * 12 hours (maximum infusion rate is 10 μg/min)

Nitrates

▶ See Chap. 6.
▶ Sublingual and IV administration have rapid onset.
▶ Mechanism of action.
  • Coronary artery vasodilation
  • Systemic vasodilation (primarily venous)
    ○ Reduces preload and afterload (to a lesser extent than preload)
▶ Potential side effects that limit usage:
  • Hypotension
  • Headache
  • Tachyphylaxis
▶ Dose (Table 11-2):

TABLE 11-2.
NITRATE DOSING IN MYOCARDIAL INFARCTION

Method of administration	Dose
Sublingual	0.4 mg q5min; may repeat 3×
Transdermal or paste	0.2–0.8 mg/hr
IV	0.1–5.0 µg/kg/min

Beta-Blockers

► See Chap. 6.
► Administer IV in the acute stage.
► Proven reduction in mortality:
  • Decreases heart rate and contractility
    ○ Decreases myocardial oxygen demand
► Potential adverse effects in the setting of an acute MI:
  • Heart failure
  • Bradycardia
  • Hypotension
  • Bronchospasm (more common with non-selective beta-blockers)

Angiotensin-Converting Enzyme Inhibitors

► Recommended within the first 24 hours of symptom onset.
  • Start with low dose, short-acting agent and titrate upward.
    ○ Captopril (Capoten): 6.25 mg PO TID
  • Decreases afterload.
► Potential limitations of usage:
  • Hypotension
  • Declining renal function

Morphine

► See Chap. 6.
► Reduces preload via venodilatation.
► Decreases pain:
  • Decreases sympathetic activity
    ○ May reduce thrombus propagation
    ○ May raise the threshold for ventricular fibrillation

Heparin

▶ Interferes with the common pathway of the coagulation cascade.
  • Inhibits additional formation and propagation of thrombi.
▶ Administer for at least 48 hours post-MI.
  • IV route ensures intended dose delivery.
  • Dose:
    ○ 60–70 units/kg IV load (maximum, 5000 units).
    ○ 12–15 units/kg/hr IV maintenance drip.
    ○ Titrate to maintain PTT 1.5–2.5 * control.
▶ Recommended for patients who undergo percutaneous revascularization or thrombolytic therapy as well.
▶ Can also administer low-molecular-weight heparin:
  • Enoxaparin (Lovenox): 1 mg/kg SC q 12 hours
  • Dalteparin (Fragmin): 120 IU/kg SC q 12 hours (maximum, 10,000 IU in 24 hours)

Revascularization Options

Thrombolytic Therapy
▶ Most effective when therapy is initiated within 30 minutes of presentation to the emergency room.
▶ Restores coronary blood flow in 50–80% of MI patients.
▶ Coadminister heparin therapy along with thrombolytics.
▶ Not indicated for patients who present more than 24 hours after symptom onset.
▶ Possible regimens
  • Alteplase (Activase, t-PA)/heparin infusion (75% successful patency at 90 minutes)
    ○ Alteplase dose
      ▪ Patient > 67 kg: 15-mg IV bolus, then 50 mg over 30 minutes, then 35 mg over next 60 minutes
      ▪ Patient ≤ 67 kg: 15-mg IV bolus, then 0.75 mg/kg over 30 minutes, then 0.5 mg/kg over next 60 minutes
  • Reteplase (Retavase)/heparin infusion (75% successful patency at 90 minutes)
    ○ Reteplase dose
      ▪ 10.8 units IV over 2 minutes
      ▪ Repeat in 30 minutes

- Streptokinase (Streptase)/heparin infusion (50% successful patency at 90 minutes)
  - Streptokinase dose
    - 1.5 million units IV over 60 minutes

Percutaneous Revascularization
▶ Most effective when therapy is initiated within 90 minutes of presentation to the emergency room
▶ Restores coronary blood flow in 90–95% of MI patients
▶ If available, it is the preferred therapy over thrombolytics
▶ Operator dependent

Surgical Revascularization
▶ Indications
  - Failed percutaneous intervention
  - Level/degree of coronary occlusion contraindicates percutaneous intervention
    - Left main coronary artery disease
    - Three-vessel disease
    - Two-vessel disease that is not amenable to a percutaneous intervention
  - Mechanical complications of MI
    - Septal defect
    - Free wall rupture
    - Acute mitral regurgitation
▶ Most useful if performed within 2–3 hours of symptom onset

Hemodynamic Considerations
▶ Maintain euvolemia.
  - May need central venous catheter or PA catheter to help guide therapy (see Chap. 5).
▶ Minimize tachycardia.
▶ When necessary, pressors to consider using include:
  - Dobutamine (see Chap. 6).
    - Has the advantage of having a minimal chronotropic effect.
    - May need to add an α-receptor agonist to counter possible systemic vasodilatation.
  - Dopamine (see Chap. 6).

- Phosphodiesterase inhibitors (see Chap. 6).
  - May need to add an α-receptor agonist to counter possible systemic vasodilatation.
▶ Intra-aortic balloon pump
- Augments both systolic and diastolic pressure using a balloon
  - Systole: balloon deflates
  - Diastole: balloon inflates (increases diastolic pressure and thus increases coronary artery perfusion)

CHAPTER 12

CONGESTIVE HEART FAILURE

ABBREVIATIONS

ACE I: angiotensin-converting enzyme inhibitor
COPD: chronic obstructive pulmonary disease
FIO_2: inspired fraction of oxygen
HR: heart rate
LV: left ventricular

DEFINITION

▶ Inadequate systemic perfusion to meet the body's requirements as a result of cardiac pump dysfunction
  • Categories
    ○ Systolic heart failure
      ▪ Reduced cardiac contractility
    ○ Diastolic heart failure
      ▪ Impaired cardiac relaxation and impaired ventricular filling
  • Types of heart failure
    ○ LV systolic dysfunction
      ▪ Most common
      ▪ Usually secondary to coronary artery disease and chronic ischemia
    ○ LV diastolic dysfunction
      ▪ Usually secondary to chronic hypertension or ischemia
    ○ Right ventricular systolic dysfunction
      ▪ Usually secondary to LV systolic dysfunction
    ○ Right ventricular diastolic dysfunction
      ▪ Consider pericardial constriction or cardiac tamponade

- Etiology of heart failure
  - Coronary artery disease
  - Chronic hypertension
  - Idiopathic dilated cardiomyopathy
  - Valvular heart disease
  - Toxin-induced cardiomyopathies
  - High cardiac output failure
  - Congenital
- ▶ New York Heart Association symptom classification system
  - Class I
    - No symptom limitation with ordinary physical activity
  - Class II
    - Ordinary physical activity slightly limited by dyspnea (e.g., long-distance walking, climbing two flights of stairs)
  - Class III
    - Mild physical activity limited by dyspnea (e.g., short-distance walking, climbing one flight of stairs)
  - Class IV
    - Dyspnea at rest or with minimal exertion

PATHOPHYSIOLOGY

- ▶ Inadequate cardiac output and systemic hypoperfusion lead to the activation of several compensatory neurohormonal pathways, which eventually become harmful to the patient.
  - Increased activity of the sympathetic nervous system
    - Increases circulating catecholamines
      - Increases HR
      - Increases contractility
      - Increases arteriolar vasoconstriction
      - Increases secretion of renin from juxtaglomerular apparatus of the kidney (see below)
      - Adverse effects
        - ➤ Predispose to dysrhythmias
        - ➤ Can worsen ischemia
        - ➤ Induce cardiac remodeling
        - ➤ Directly toxic to myocytes

- Increased activity of the renin-angiotensin system
  - Increases arteriolar vasoconstriction
  - Increases release of aldosterone
    - Increases sodium and water retention
    - Leads to endothelial dysfunction
    - Leads to organ fibrosis
- Increased baroreceptor activity
  - Stimulates release of vasopressin (antidiuretic hormone) from the hypothalamus
    - Increases water reabsorption
▶ Increased release of natriuretic peptides from cardiac myocytes provides a counter-regulatory effort:
  - Increases systemic vasodilation
  - Increases pulmonary vasodilation
  - Increases sodium and water excretion

Note: Neurohormonal stimulation leads to LV remodeling, specifically dilatation and hypertrophy. These changes can cause increased wall tension, worsen myocardial perfusion, worsen mitral regurgitation, potentiate cardiac ischemia, and even lead to myocardial cell death.

SYMPTOMS AND SIGNS

Symptoms

▶ Dyspnea with exertion or at rest
▶ Orthopnea
▶ Paroxysmal nocturnal dyspnea
▶ Fatigue
▶ Cachexia

Signs

▶ Tachycardia
▶ Tachypnea
▶ Bilateral inspiratory rales
▶ Hypoxia
▶ Jugular venous distention

► Peripheral edema
► Hepatosplenomegaly
► Ascites
► Auscultation of heart sounds
  • Presence of an S_3 and/or S_4 heart sound
  • Murmurs of mitral and/or tricuspid insufficiency

DIAGNOSIS

► History and physical exam
► Electrocardiogram
  • Rhythm
    ○ Normal, sinus tachycardia, or atrial fibrillation
  • LV hypertrophy, left bundle branch block, intraventricular conduction delay, and nonspecific ST-segment and T-wave changes
► Chest radiograph
  • Cardiomegaly
  • Pulmonary venous congestion
  • Kerley B lines
  • Alveolar edema
  • Pleural effusions
► Echocardiography
  • Differentiates between systolic and diastolic dysfunction
  • Provides information about chamber size, severity of hypertrophy, and valvular function
► Serum B-type natriuretic peptide (BNP) measurement
  • < 100 pg/ml
    ○ Patient is not likely in heart failure
  • > 100 pg/ml
    ○ Suggests that patient is in heart failure
    ○ Differentiates from COPD exacerbation
    ○ Serum levels correlate with the severity of heart failure

Note: These values may differ for individual laboratories.

MANAGEMENT

Airway

► Ensure stable airway.
  • Consider mechanical ventilation if necessary (see Chap. 4).

Breathing

▶ Optimize oxygenation (see Chap. 3).
  • Increase FIO_2.
  • Consider mechanical ventilation if necessary (see Chap. 4).

Goal

▶ The basis of current therapy is aimed at countering the potentially harmful compensatory efforts of the neurohormonal pathways.

Nonpharmacologic Therapy

▶ Dietary sodium restriction
▶ Fluid restriction

Pharmacotherapy

Angiotensin-Converting Enzyme Inhibitors

▶ Proven mortality benefit.
▶ Provide neurohormonal modulation.
  • Decrease angiotensin II levels.
  • Decrease angiotensin-mediated aldosterone release.
▶ Provide afterload reduction.
▶ Potential side effects:
  • Cough
  • Angioedema
  • Acute renal failure (in the setting of bilateral renal stenosis)
  • May necessitate switching to angiotensin II receptor blockers or a combination of hydralazine and nitrates to provide afterload reduction
▶ Dose:
  • Start with low-dose, short-acting agent [captopril (Capoten)] and titrate to the maximum tolerated dose.
  • Can switch to a long-acting agent [lisinopril (Zestril), enalapril (Vasotec)] once stable dose is achieved.
  • Target doses
    ○ Captopril: 50 mg PO TID
    ○ Lisinopril: 40 mg PO QD
    ○ Enalapril: 20 mg PO BID or 0.625–2.50 mg IV q 6 hours

Angiotensin II Receptor Blockers
► Proven mortality benefit, but not better than ACE I
► Second-line therapy for patients who are intolerant to ACE I due to cough or angioedema
► Dose
- Irbesartan (Avapro): 75–300 mg PO QD
- Losartan (Cozaar): 50–100 mg PO QD
- Valsartan (Diovan): 80–320 mg PO QD

Beta-Blockers
► Proven mortality benefit.
► Reduce myocardial oxygen consumption by decreasing heart rate.
► Can potentially worsen acute failure.
► Dose:
- Initiate with a very low dose and slowly titrate upward.
- Carvedilol (Coreg): 3.125–25.0 mg PO BID (may go up to 50 mg PO BID for patients > 75 kg).

Digoxin
► No effect on mortality
► Weak oral inotrope
► Provides neurohormonal modulation
► Dose
- 0.125–0.375 mg PO/IV QD (use loading dose of 0.5 mg for IV route)

Aldosterone Antagonists
► Proven mortality benefit
► Potassium-sparing diuretic effect
- Monitor potassium levels to avoid hyperkalemia
- Avoid in patients with renal dysfunction
► Dose
- Spironolactone (Aldactone): 12.5–50 mg PO QD
- Eplerenone (Inspra): 25–50 mg PO QD

Diuretics
► Loop diuretics
- No proven mortality benefit
- Provide symptomatic relief and improve oxygenation

- Dose
  - Furosemide (Lasix): 10–40 mg PO/IV q 6 hours – QD (equivalent PO dose is two times IV dose)
  - Bumetanide (Bumex): 0.5–1.0 mg PO/IV QD
  - Torsemide (Demadex): 5–20 mg PO/IV QD
  - Ethacrynic acid (Edecrin): 0.5–1.0 mg/kg IV QD or 25–100 mg PO QD/BID (mainly used if patient is allergic to furosemide)
- ▶ Thiazide diuretics
  - No proven mortality benefit
  - Second-line agents to loop diuretics
  - Dose
    - Hydrochlorothiazide (HCTZ): 12.5–50 mg PO QD
    - Metolazone (Zaroxolyn): 5–20 mg PO QD

Intravenous Inotropes and Vasodilators
- ▶ Dobutamine (see Chap. 6)
  - Titrate to the lowest dose that provides hemodynamic stability to minimize arrhythmogenic effect.
- ▶ Phosphodiesterase inhibitors (milrinone) (see Chap. 6)
  - Titrate to the lowest dose that provides hemodynamic stability to minimize arrhythmogenic effect.
- ▶ Nitroglycerin (see Chap. 6)
  - Predominant benefit is from pre-load reduction and coronary artery vasodilation
  - Usage limited by hypotension
- ▶ Sodium nitroprusside (see Chap. 6)
  - Predominant benefit is from pre-load and afterload reduction
  - Usage limited by hypotension
  - Should be avoided in patients with active cardiac ischemia due to the potential of "coronary steal," which shunts blood away from ischemic myocardium to well-perfused areas
- ▶ Nesiritide (Natrecor)
  - Synthetic BNP
  - Arterial and venous vasodilator
    - Increases cardiac output
    - Does not increase heart rate
  - Modest diuretic and natriuretic effect
  - Dose
    - 2 µg/kg IV bolus then 0.01 µg/kg/min IV infusion

Invasive Therapies

- ▶ Biventricular pacing
  - Improves synchronization of ventricular contraction
    - ○ Optimized with echocardiographic guidance
  - Reduces severity of mitral regurgitation
- ▶ LV assist device (LVAD)
  - Consider in patients who are unresponsive to inotrope and intra-aortic balloon pump therapy
  - Mainly used as a bridge to cardiac transplantation
- ▶ Cardiac transplantation

CHAPTER 13

CHRONIC OBSTRUCTIVE PULMONARY DISEASE EXACERBATION

ABBREVIATIONS

COPD: chronic obstructive pulmonary disease
FEV_1: forced expiratory volume in 1 second
FVC: forced vital capacity
MDI: metered-dose inhaler
$PaCO_2$: partial pressure of carbon dioxide (mmHg) – arterial
PaO_2: partial pressure of oxygen (mmHg) – arterial
SaO_2: arterial oxygen saturation

DEFINITION

► Chronic, progressive airflow obstruction that consists of a large irreversible component
► Two main categories
   • Emphysema (pink puffer)
      ○ Alveolar wall destruction with enlargement of air spaces distal to the terminal bronchioles and without evidence of fibrosis
   • Chronic bronchitis (blue bloater)
      ○ Productive cough that is present for a period of 3 months in each of 2 consecutive years in the absence of another cause of excessive sputum production

PATHOPHYSIOLOGY

Emphysema

► Elastin breakdown resulting in destruction of alveolar walls
   • Mainly caused by cigarette smoke

- • Neutrophil-mediated inflammatory process
- ► Oxidative stress
- ► Imbalance of protease/anti-protease activity
  - • Predisposes to pan-acinar form of emphysema (α_1-antitrypsin deficiency)

Chronic Bronchitis

- ► Hallmark is an increase in goblet size and number
  - • Leads to excessive mucus secretion

SYMPTOMS AND SIGNS

Symptoms

- ► Cough
- ► Dyspnea
- ► Increased sputum production

Signs

- ► Wheezing
- ► Prolonged expiration
  - • Pursed-lip breathing
- ► Barrel chest
- ► Use of accessory muscles of breathing
- ► Hypercapnia
- ► Hypoxia
- ► Altered mental status
- ► Evidence of right heart failure (seen in severe cases – secondary to chronic pulmonary hypertension)
  - • Peripheral edema

DIAGNOSIS

History and Physical Examination

- ► Main diagnostic tool when patients present to the emergency room with an acute exacerbation

Spirometry

▶ Decreased FEV_1
  - 50–80% predicted: mild
  - 35–49% predicted: moderate
  - < 35% predicted: severe
▶ Decreased FEV_1/FVC ratio
  - Normal ratio is 70–75% in healthy lungs
  - In COPD, both FEV_1 and FVC are decreased, but the FEV_1 is affected more which results in a decreased ratio
    ◦ Ratio < 70–75% suggests COPD
▶ Many patients will have evidence of a reversible airflow obstruction as demonstrated by improved spirometry after bronchodilator therapy

Diffusing Capacity for Carbon Monoxide (DLCO)

▶ Reduced alveolar-capillary units result in a decreased diffusing capacity for carbon monoxide
  - Suggestive of emphysema

Chest X-Ray

▶ Hyperinflation
▶ Flattening of the diaphragms
▶ Peripheral bullae and blebs

MANAGEMENT

Airway

▶ Ensure secure airway.
  - Consider mechanical ventilation if necessary (see Chap. 4)

Oxygen Therapy

▶ Maintain PaO_2 approximately 60–65 mmHg.
  - Do not need to maintain an SaO_2 of 100% as this can potentially blunt the "hypoxic drive to breath" that can develop in COPD patients due to their chronic state of hypercapnia (elevated $PaCO_2$).

▶ Consider noninvasive positive pressure ventilation or mechanical ventilation if necessary (see Chap. 4).

Bronchodilators

▶ β_2-Adrenergic agonists
  - Albuterol (Ventolin)
    ◦ May have side effect of tachycardia due to β_1-agonist properties
    ◦ Dose
      ▪ MDI 2–4 puffs q 4–6 hours
      ▪ Nebulized treatment q 4–6 hours
▶ Anticholinergic therapy
  - Ipratropium bromide (Atrovent)
    ◦ Dose
      ▪ MDI 2 puffs q 4–6 hours
      ▪ Nebulized treatment q 4–6 hours
▶ Combination therapy
  - Albuterol/ipratropium (Combivent)
    ◦ Dose
      ▪ MDI 2 puffs q 4–6 hours
▶ Consider IV aminophylline if inadequate response to the above (rarely used)
    ◦ Dose
      ▪ Load 6 mg/kg IV over 30 minutes, then 0.5–0.7 mg/kg/hr

Chest Physiotherapy

▶ Recommended by American Thoracic Society only if sputum volume is > 25 ml/day

Antibiotics

▶ Start with narrow-spectrum antibiotic.
  - Coverage should include *Streptococcus pneumoniae, Haemophilus influenzae,* and *Moraxella catarrhalis.*
    ◦ Consider amoxicillin, doxycycline, or levofloxacin.
▶ Duration of therapy: 7–14 days.
▶ Broaden coverage if no response.

Corticosteroids

► Oral therapy
  • Prednisone
    ○ Start with high dose therapy and titrate down.
    ○ 60 → 5 mg PO QD.
► Systemic (IV) therapy
  • Methylprednisolone (Solu-Medrol)
    ○ Start with high dose therapy and titrate down.
    ○ 250 → 10 mg IV QD.
      ▪ Higher doses can be administered as divided doses.
► Duration of therapy: 5–10 days.

Noninvasive Positive Pressure or Mechanical Ventilation

► Noninvasive positive pressure (see Chap. 4)
  • Improves oxygenation and ventilation
  • Reduces the need for intubation
  • Proven mortality benefit
  • Contraindications
    ○ Altered mental status
    ○ Inadequate mask application
    ○ Hemodynamic instability
► Mechanical ventilation (see Chap. 4)

CHAPTER 14

COMMUNITY- AND HOSPITAL-ACQUIRED PNEUMONIA

ABBREVIATIONS

CAP: community-acquired pneumonia
CXR: chest x-ray
FIO$_2$: inspired fraction of oxygen
HAP: hospital-acquired pneumonia
ICU: intensive care unit
TBA: tracheobronchial aspirate

DEFINITION

Community-Acquired Pneumonia

► Pneumonia acquired outside of hospitals or extended-care facilities

Hospital-Acquired Pneumonia

► Pneumonia acquired in the hospital setting
► Begins > 48 hours after admission to the hospital
► Most common infection in patients in the ICU
  • Usually selects for in-hospital organisms
    ○ Gram-negative organisms
    ○ Resistant strains
► More common in mechanically ventilated patients
  • Endotracheal tube bypasses upper respiratory tract defenses.
  • Predisposes to pooling of oropharyngeal secretions.
  • Prevents cough.
  • Foreign object can be a nidus for infection.

PATHOPHYSIOLOGY

Mechanisms/Risk Factors of Acquiring Infection

▶ Inhalation of infectious particles
  - Most common route for CAP
▶ Microaspiration/aspiration
  - Most common route for HAP
    ◦ Contaminated oropharyngeal secretions.
      ▪ Thirty-five percent to 70% of hospitalized patients have oropharyngeal secretions colonized with gram-negative bacteria.
    ◦ Endotracheal and nasogastric tubes interfere with anatomic defenses.
  - Less common route for CAP
    ◦ Microaspiration is usually benign
      ▪ Occurs in up to 50% of sleeping individuals
▶ Direct inoculation
  - Tracheobronchial tree deposition
    ◦ Examples include from surgery and bronchoscopy
    ◦ Less common route
  - Hematogenous deposition
    ◦ Uncommon route
▶ Direct extension of infection from anatomically contiguous areas
  - Examples include pleural or subdiaphragmatic spaces
  - Rare
▶ Reactivation of preexisting pathogens
  - Examples include *Pneumocystis carinii, Mycobacterium tuberculosis,* and cytomegalovirus.
  - More common in immunocompromised patients.
▶ Defects in defenses
  - Impaired local pulmonary defenses
    ◦ Impaired cough reflex
      ▪ Stroke
      ▪ Sedatives
      ▪ Poor nutrition
      ▪ Surgery (splinting and pain)
    ◦ Impaired mucociliary transport
      ▪ Smoking

- Increased age
- Dehydration
- Impaired cellular and humoral immune response
  - Increased age
  - Diabetes mellitus
  - Poor nutrition
  - Corticosteroids
  - Hypothermia
  - Hypophosphatemia
  - Chemotherapy
  - Hematologic malignancy
  - Human immunodeficiency virus

Microbiology

Community-Acquired Pneumonia
▶ Gram-positive bacteria
  - Most common
    - *Streptococcus pneumoniae*
▶ Gram-negative bacteria
  - Less common
    - *Haemophilus influenzae, Klebsiella pneumoniae, Moraxella catarrhalis, Legionella* species
  - Can be seen with greater frequency in smokers
▶ Atypical pneumonia
  - Less common
    - *Mycoplasma pneumoniae, Chlamydia pneumoniae*

Hospital-Acquired Pneumonia
▶ Gram-negative bacteria
  - Most common (55–85% causative organism)
  - Consider other organisms along with those typically seen with CAP
    - *Pseudomonas aeruginosa, Escherichia coli, Acinetobacter* species, *Enterobacter* species, *Proteus* species, *Serratia marcescens*
▶ Gram-positive bacteria
  - Less common
    - Consider methicillin-resistant *Staphylococcus aureus* (MRSA)

▶ Anaerobic bacteria
- Rarely associated with aspiration events (usually < 5–10% of the time)
    ◦ Unusual except when associated with lung abscesses
    ◦ Consider *Bacteroides* species

SYMPTOMS AND SIGNS

Symptoms

▶ Productive cough
▶ Fever and/or chills
▶ Dyspnea

Signs

▶ Fever
▶ Tachypnea
▶ Tachycardia
▶ Hypoxia
▶ Decreased breath sounds, usually localized to a specific lung zone
▶ Dullness to percussion, usually localized to a specific lung zone

DIAGNOSIS

▶ History and physical examination
▶ Laboratory blood test
- White blood cell count
    ◦ Leukocytosis or leukopenia
- Serologic testing
    ◦ Available for *Legionella*, *Mycoplasma*, and *Chlamydia*
    ◦ Usually reserved for patients with the appropriate history and physical findings to suggest these pathogens
▶ CXR
- Infiltrate, usually confined to a specific lung zone
▶ Sputum Gram stain and culture
- Poor sensitivity and specificity
    ◦ Often contaminated with oropharyngeal secretions

- ○ Poor method for identifying pathogen
  - Specimen should have < 10 epithelial cells
► Tracheobronchial aspirate (TBA)
  - Good sensitivity
  - Most useful noninvasive test
  - Cannot distinguish between colonizers and pathogen
    - ○ Best used to exclude resistant organisms, which helps guide the narrowing of antibiotic coverage
► Blood culture
  - Obtain before administering antibiotics
  - Poor sensitivity and specificity
  - Has mostly a prognostic value
► Invasive bronchoscopic testing
  - Methods
    - ○ Bronchoalveolar lavage
    - ○ Protected brush catheter
    - ○ Transbronchial biopsy
  - Similar sensitivity and specificity as TBA
  - No proven mortality benefit
  - Usually reserved for deteriorating patients without an etiologic diagnosis
► Tissue culture and histology testing
  - Methods
    - ○ Thorascopic lung biopsy
    - ○ Open lung biopsy
  - Reserved for deteriorating patients in whom bronchoscopic techniques failed to provide a diagnosis

MANAGEMENT

Airway

► Ensure stable airway.
  - Consider mechanical ventilation if necessary (see Chap. 4).

Oxygenation

► Optimize oxygenation (see Chap. 3).
  - Increase FIO_2.
  - Consider mechanical ventilation if necessary (see Chap. 4).

Antimicrobial Therapy

Community-Acquired Pneumonia
▶ Begin with empiric therapy that covers the usual organisms.
- Macrolide plus ceftriaxone/cefotaxime
- Fluoroquinolone plus ceftriaxone/cefotaxime
- Beta lactam/beta lactamase inhibitor
▶ If the patient does not respond, consider additional testing such as TBA or bronchoscopic techniques to identify the pathogen and guide further antimicrobial therapy.

Hospital-Acquired Pneumonia
▶ Avoid monotherapy for severe HAP that requires ICU care.
▶ Begin with empiric therapy that covers the usual organisms.
- Fluoroquinolone plus ceftriaxone/cefuroxime
- Fluoroquinolone plus beta lactam/beta lactamase inhibitor
- Fluoroquinolone alone (less severe HAP)
▶ For patients with suspected aspiration, consider covering anaerobes.
- Clindamycin
- Metronidazole
- Beta lactam/beta lactamase inhibitor
- Second-generation cephalosporin
  - Cefmetazole
  - Cefoxitin
  - Cefotetan
▶ For patients with suspected *S. aureus* infection.
- Vancomycin
  - Covers methicillin-resistant *S. aureus* until sensitivities are known.
    - Change to oxacillin if the pathogen is sensitive.
  - Titrate dose to peak/trough levels.
▶ For patients with a prolonged ICU course (> 5 days), cover *P. aeruginosa.*
- Ciprofloxacin
- Gentamicin
- Ceftazidime
- Piperacillin/tazobactam
- Imipenem or meropenem

Duration of Therapy
▶ No consensus regarding the correct duration of therapy.
▶ Duration should be titrated to the patient's clinical response.
▶ Usual course is 7–14 days.

Doses of Commonly Used Antibiotics
▶ Aminoglycosides
  • Gentamicin (Garamycin): 1 mg/kg IV/IM q 8 hours or 4–6 mg/kg IV QD
    ○ Titrate to peak/trough levels to avoid nephrotoxicity.
      ▪ Peak: 5–10 µg/ml
      ▪ Trough: 0.1–2.0 µg/ml
▶ Carbapenems
  • Imipenem (Primaxin): 250–1000 mg IV q 6–8 hours
  • Meropenem (Merrem): 1 g IV q 8 hours
▶ Cephalosporins
  • Cefotetan (Cefotan): 1–2 g IV/IM q 12 hours
  • Cefoxitin (Mefoxin): 1–2 g IV/IM q 6–8 hours
  • Cefuroxime (Ceftin): 750–1500 mg IV/IM q 8 hours
  • Ceftazidime (Fortaz): 1–2 g IV q 8–12 hours
  • Ceftriaxone (Rocephin): 1–2 g IV/IM QD
▶ Fluoroquinolones
  • Levofloxacin (Levaquin): 250–500 mg IV/PO QD
  • Ciprofloxacin (Cipro): 200–400 mg IV q 12 hours or 250–750 mg PO q 12 hours
▶ Macrolides
  • Azithromycin (Zithromax): 500 mg IV QD
  • Clarithromycin (Biaxin): 250–500 mg PO q 12 hours
▶ Beta lactam/beta lactamase inhibitors
  • Ampicillin/sulbactam (Unasyn): 1.5–3.0 g IV/IM q 6 hours
  • Piperacillin/tazobactam (Zosyn): 2.25–4.5 g IV q 4–6 hours
▶ Others
  • Aztreonam (Azactam): 0.5–2.0 g IV/IM q 6–12 hours
  • Clindamycin (Cleocin): 600–900 mg IV q 8 hours
  • Metronidazole (Flagyl): 500 mg IV/PO q 8 hours
  • Vancomycin (Vancocin): 1 g IV q 12 hours
    ○ Titrate to peak/trough levels to avoid nephrotoxicity.
      ▪ Peak: 20–40 µg/ml
      ▪ Trough: 5–15 µg/ml

○ Recently, the utility and significance of serum levels have been questioned.

Note: Many of the antibiotic doses need to be adjusted for renal dysfunction as measured by a declining creatinine clearance (ml/min).

CHAPTER 15

SEPSIS

ABBREVIATIONS

ACTH: adrenocorticotropic hormone
APC: activated protein C
ARDS: acute respiratory distress syndrome
BP: blood pressure
CNS: central nervous system
CVP: central venous pressure
DVT: deep venous thrombosis
FIO_2: inspired fraction of oxygen
IL: interleukin
INR: international normalized ratio
MAP: mean arterial pressure
PA: pulmonary artery
PaO_2: partial pressure of oxygen (mmHg) – arterial
PCWP: pulmonary capillary wedge pressure
SIRS: systemic inflammatory response syndrome
TNF-α: tumor necrosis factor alpha
WBC: white blood cell

DEFINITION

▶ Systemic inflammatory response syndrome (SIRS)
  • Patient's response to illness of either infectious or non-infectious (e.g., trauma, burns, pancreatitis) etiology that consists of
    ◦ Core temperature alterations
      ▪ Hyperthermia
      ▪ Hypothermia
    ◦ Tachycardia
    ◦ Tachypnea

- ○ WBC count alterations
  - ▪ Leukocytosis
  - ▪ Leukopenia
- ▶ Sepsis
  - • SIRS secondary to a known or presumed site of infection
- ▶ Septic shock
  - • Sepsis that results in hypotension and inadequate end-organ perfusion

PATHOPHYSIOLOGY

Initiation of the Inflammatory Cascade

- ▶ Bacteria are the most common cause by way of components of the outer membrane
  - • Gram-negative organisms
    - ○ Lipopolysaccharide, lipid A, endotoxin
  - • Gram-positive organisms
    - ○ Lipoteichoic acid, peptidoglycan
- ▶ Fungi, viruses, and parasites can also cause sepsis

Inflammation Leads to the Production of Proinflammatory Cytokines

- ▶ TNF-α
- ▶ IL-1
  - • Direct cytotoxic effects
  - • Promote nitric oxide synthase activity
    - ○ Can lead to vasodilatation and hypotension
  - • Promote neutrophil activity

Inflammation Leads to Coagulation

- ▶ IL-1 and TNF-α have direct effects on the endothelial surface
  - • Increase the expression of tissue factor
    - ○ Activates extrinsic pathway of coagulation
      - ▪ Increases the production of thrombin
        - ➢ Increases the formation of fibrin clots in the microvasculature
- ▶ IL-1 and TNF-α increase the production of plasminogen activator inhibitor-1
  - • Inhibits fibrinolysis

▶ Proinflammatory cytokines (e.g., IL-1, TNF-α) impair the activation of naturally occurring modulators of inflammation and coagulation

▶ Activated protein C (APC)
- Normal functions
  - Activated in the presence of thrombin and thrombomodulin
  - Inhibits thrombin production (along with cofactor protein S)
  - Inhibits plasminogen activator inhibitor-1
    - Restores fibrinolytic function
  - Has direct antiinflammatory properties
    - Decreases production of proinflammatory cytokines
    - Inhibits neutrophil adhesion and accumulation
- Proinflammatory cytokines *prevent* the activation of protein C

▶ Antithrombin
- Normal functions.
  - Inhibits thrombin production.
  - When bound to endothelial cell surface glycosaminoglycans, leads to the production of the anti-inflammatory molecule prostacyclin (PGI$_2$).
- Neutrophil-mediated elastase cleaves glycosaminoglycans off the surface and, thus, limits the antiinflammatory effects of antithrombin.

Final Common Pathway

▶ Cardiovascular insufficiency
- Myocardial-depressant effects of TNF-α
- Systemic vasodilatation leading to hypotension
- Capillary leak
▶ End-organ hypoperfusion leading to multiple organ failure
- Often leads to death

SYMPTOMS AND SIGNS

Symptoms

▶ Fever
▶ Chills

- ▶ Diaphoresis
- ▶ Vertigo or syncope
- ▶ Variable symptoms depending on etiology of sepsis
  - • Productive cough and dyspnea (pneumonia)
  - • Dysuria, increased frequency of urination, suprapubic or flank pain (urosepsis)
  - • Abdominal pain (abdominal source of sepsis)

Signs

- ▶ Temperature alteration
  - • Hyperthermia
  - • Hypothermia
- ▶ Tachycardia
- ▶ Tachypnea
- ▶ Mental status changes
- ▶ Laboratory tests
  - • WBC count
    - ○ Leukocytosis
    - ○ Leukopenia
  - • Unexplained impairment in renal or liver function
  - • Lactic acidosis
  - • Elevated C-reactive protein

DIAGNOSIS

- ▶ Presumed or known site of infection:
  - • Pneumonia
  - • Gastrointestinal (e.g., appendicitis, cholecystitis, diverticulitis, bowel perforation)
  - • Urinary tract infection/pyelonephritis
  - • Abscess or infected collection
  - • Positive blood cultures (from a known or unknown site)
  - • Infected mechanical hardware
- ▶ Evidence of SIRS as indicated by the presence of at least two of the following:
  - • Core temperature alteration
    - ○ Fever ($\geq 38^{\circ}$C, 100.4°F)
    - ○ Hypothermia ($\leq 36^{\circ}$C, 96.8°F)
  - • Tachypnea
  - • Tachycardia

- WBC count alteration
  - Leukocytosis ($\geq$ 12,000 cells/mm^3)
  - Leukopenia ($\leq$ 4000 cells/mm^3)
  - Bandemia ($\geq$ 10% bands on differential)
- ▶ Evidence of sepsis-induced organ failure:
  - Cardiovascular
    - MAP $\leq$ 60 mmHg in the setting of normal to elevated cardiac output (measured by PA catheter)
    - Need for vasopressors to maintain adequate BP in the setting of adequate intravascular volume
  - Respiratory
    - PaO$_2$/FIO$_2$ ratio < 250 in the absence of pneumonia
    - PaO$_2$/FIO$_2$ ratio < 200 in the presence of pneumonia
  - Renal
    - Urine output < 0.5 ml/kg/hr for 1 hour in the setting of adequate intravascular volume
  - Hematologic
    - INR > 1.2 otherwise not explained by liver disease or warfarin usage
  - Metabolic acidosis
    - Acidemia with a pH < 7.30 and a plasma lactate level > 1.5 times the normal laboratory value

MANAGEMENT

Airway

- ▶ Ensure a stable airway.
  - Consider mechanical ventilation if necessary (see Chap. 4).

Oxygenation

- ▶ Optimize oxygenation (see Chap. 3).
  - Increase FIO$_2$.
  - Consider mechanical ventilation if necessary (see Chap. 4).

Antimicrobial Therapy

- ▶ Begin with broad-spectrum empiric therapy that covers the usual causative organisms.
  - Gram positive
    - *Staphylococcus aureus*

- ○ *Streptococcus pneumoniae*
- Gram negative
  - ○ *Escherichia coli*
  - ○ *Klebsiella* species
▶ Specific considerations:
  - If nosocomial pneumonia is suspected
    - ○ Cover *Pseudomonas* and *Enterobacter* species.
  - If intra-abdominal source is suspected
    - ○ Cover enteric gram-negative and anaerobic organisms.
    - ○ Cover *Enterococcus* species.
      - ▪ Two main species to consider
        - ➤ *E. faecalis* (more common)
          - ❖ Usually treated with ampicillin or levofloxacin
        - ➤ *E. faecium* (less common)
          - ❖ Can develop vancomycin/levofloxacin resistance
          - ❖ Usually treated with ampicillin
  - If prosthetic device infection is suspected
    - ○ Cover gram-negative and gram-positive organisms (including *Enterococcus*).
    - ○ Consider administering vancomycin to empirically cover methicillin-resistant *S. aureus* and methicillin-resistant *Staphylococcus epidermidis* (MRSE) until sensitivities are known.

Empiric Antifungal Therapy

▶ Consider only for patients at higher risk for fungemia
  - Fungal colonization at two or more sites
  - Already received > 14 days of antibiotic therapy
  - Upper gastrointestinal (stomach, duodenum) perforation
  - Chronic steroid therapy
  - Chronic total parenteral nutrition therapy
▶ Medications
  - Fluconazole (Diflucan)
    - ○ Dose: 200–400 mg IV/PO QD
  - Caspofungin (Cancidas)
    - ○ Dose: 70-mg IV loading dose, then 50 mg IV QD
    - ○ Consider for fluconazole-resistant *Candida* species

- Amphotericin B (Fungizone)
  - Test dose: 0.1 mg/kg to 1 mg IV once
    - Wait 2–4 hours to see if patient tolerates
  - Dose: 0.25–1.5 mg/kg IV QD
  - Monitor for nephrotoxicity
- Liposomal amphotericin B (AmBisome)
  - Dose: 3–5 mg/kg IV QD given over 2 hours
  - Less nephrotoxic
- Voriconazole (Vfend)
  - Dose:
    - IV: 6 mg/kg q 12 hours × 2 doses, then 4 mg/kg q 12 hours
    - PO: 200 mg q 12 hours if > 40 kg, 100 mg q 12 hours if < 40 kg

Infection Control

▶ Control the source of infection.
- Consider removing infected foreign bodies.
  - Urinary catheters
  - Intravascular catheters
  - Prosthetic joints
  - Vascular grafts
- Incision and drainage of abscesses/infected collections.
- Surgical débridement/resection of infected/necrotic tissue or viscera.

Cardiovascular Support

▶ IV fluid resuscitation
- Most patients require an aggressive fluid challenge.
- Minimizes a pre-renal component of renal insufficiency.
- Titrate fluid resuscitation to filling pressure measurements.
  - Central venous catheter
    - CVP 10–12 mmHg
  - PA catheter (see Chap. 5)
    - PCWP 18 mmHg
  - Can also help guide vasopressor therapy
▶ Vasopressor therapy
- Main goals:
  - Increase systemic vascular tone.

- ○ Optimize cardiac output and delivery of oxygen to peripheral tissues (see Chap. 3).
- Consider the following regimens (see Chap. 6):
    - ○ Norepinephrine (Levophed) ± vasopressin
        - Consider as the first choice
        - May add dopamine if the patient remains hypotensive on maximum doses of norepinephrine and vasopressin
    - ○ Dopamine ± vasopressin
        - Use higher doses of dopamine to target all receptors (including α and β receptors).
        - Do *not* use "renal-dose dopamine" range.
    - ○ Dobutamine ± phenylephrine (Neo-Synephrine) ± vasopressin

Acute Respiratory Distress Syndrome

▶ If the patient develops ARDS
- Institute mechanical ventilation (see Chap. 4, Chap. 19).
- Consider specific ARDS therapeutic strategies (see Chap. 19).

Glucose

▶ Correct metabolic/serum glucose abnormalities
- Maintain serum glucose ≤ 120 mg/dl

Renal Failure

▶ Consider instituting hemodialysis or continuous venovenous hemofiltration (CVVH) in patients with renal failure unresponsive to IV fluid therapy or severe metabolic derangements.

Nutrition

▶ Administer early nutrition (see Chap. 9).
- Use the parenteral route if enteral feeding is not possible.

Steroid Therapy

▶ Patients that are unresponsive to fluid resuscitation and pressor therapy may have relative adrenal insufficiency.

▶ Consider administering ACTH stimulation test to assess adrenal function, especially in patients requiring pressor support for > 72 hours:
- Measure baseline serum cortisol level (time 0).
- Administer 250 µg IV of ACTH.
- Measure serum cortisol level after 30 minutes of ACTH dose (time 1).
- Measure serum cortisol level after 60 minutes of ACTH dose (time 2).

▶ Normal response is a rise of > 9 mg/dl in the serum cortisol level by 60 minutes after ACTH administration.

▶ If the patient is adrenally hyporesponsive, consider administering the following:
- Hydrocortisone (Solu-Cortef), 50 mg IV q 6 hours for 7 days
- Fludrocortisone (Florinef), 50 µg PO/NG QD for 7 days

▶ Studies have shown improved survival compared to placebo in patients with septic shock refractory to fluids and pressor therapy and adrenal hyporesponsiveness

Recombinant Human Activated Protein C

▶ Alternate names: rhAPC, drotrecogin alfa, APC, Xigris
▶ Therapeutic properties:
- Antiinflammatory
- Anti-thrombotic
- Profibrinolytic

▶ Studies have shown mortality benefit compared to placebo.
▶ Indications:
- Evidence of septic shock (see Diagnosis section)
  ○ Presumed or known site of infection
  ○ Evidence of SIRS
  ○ Sepsis-induced organ failure
▶ Contraindications:
- Evidence of internal, gastrointestinal, or postoperative bleeding
- Surgery in the previous 12 hours
- Thrombocytopenia (≤ 20,000 platelets/mm^3)
- History of CNS mass lesion or evidence of cerebral herniation
- History of stroke, arteriovenous malformation, cerebral aneurysm, intracranial or intraspinal surgery, or severe head trauma within the last 3 months

- History of cirrhosis with portal hypertension and esophageal varices
- Nephrostomy tubes in place
- Therapeutic doses of heparin ($\geq$ 15,000 U/day) within the previous 8 hours or therapeutic doses of low-molecular-weight heparins within the previous 12 hours
- Systemic thrombolytic therapy within the past 3 days
- Anti-platelet medications within the previous 3–4 days
- Warfarin within the past 4 days
- Presence of pulmonary, liver, or splenic contusions/lacerations following trauma
- Presence of an epidural catheter

▶ Dosing guidelines:
  - 24 µg/kg/hr as a continuous infusion for 96 hours.
  - Stop infusion 2 hours before an invasive procedure.
  - May restart infusion 1 hour after a percutaneous procedure or 12 hours after a surgical procedure if adequate hemostasis has been achieved.
  - Stop infusion with any evidence of bleeding.
  - Administer stress ulcer prophylaxis.
  - Stop infusion if the patient requires therapeutic heparin for a thrombotic event.
  - If the patient requires hemodialysis, attempt to run the dialysis with APC alone or the lowest dose of heparin necessary to prevent clotting.

Additional Treatments

▶ Administer DVT prophylaxis (see Chap. 10).
▶ Administer stress ulcer prophylaxis (see Chap. 10).

CHAPTER 16

SEVERE ACUTE PANCREATITIS

ABBREVIATIONS

ALT: alanine aminotransferase
ARDS: acute respiratory distress syndrome
5-ASA: 5-aminosalicyclic acid
BUN: blood urea nitrogen
CT: computerized tomography
CVP: central venous pressure
DVT: deep venous thrombosis
ERCP: endoscopic retrograde cholangiopancreatography
FIO_2: inspired fraction of oxygen
IL: interleukin
PA: pulmonary artery
PaO_2: partial pressure of oxygen (mmHg) – arterial
PCWP: pulmonary capillary wedge pressure
TNF-α: tumor necrosis factor alpha

DEFINITION

▶ Inflammatory condition of the pancreas that consists of:
  • Abdominal pain
  • Elevated levels of pancreatic enzymes in the blood
  • Most often nonprogressive
    ○ Pancreas returns to normal function and histology after recovery if the patient survives (excludes patients with chronic pancreatitis).
▶ Inflammatory process may involve peripancreatic tissues and/ or other organ systems.

▶ *Severe* pancreatitis is characterized by one or more of the following:
- Presence of organ failure
  - Cardiovascular collapse (shock)
  - Pulmonary insufficiency
  - Renal failure
- Presence of local complications
  - Pancreatic necrosis
  - Pancreatic abscess
  - Pancreatic pseudocyst

PATHOPHYSIOLOGY

Localized to the Pancreas

▶ Premature intra-acinar activation of pancreatic proenzymes (normally stored in an inactive form)
- Proenzymes prematurely exposed to lysosomal enzymes such as cathepsin B
  - Activates trypsinogen (inactive zymogen) to trypsin (active enzyme).
  - Trypsin initiates premature activation of other pancreatic proenzymes.
  - Leads to pancreatic autodigestion.
    - Damages acinar cells
    - Damages pancreatic interstitium
    - Damages vascular endothelium
      - ➢ May contribute to intrapancreatic hemorrhage
▶ Alterations in the permeability of pancreatic ducts (primarily alcohol induced)
- Leads to the precipitation of proteinaceous plugs in the small pancreatic ductules
  - Direct toxic effect to the pancreas
  - Increased pressure from obstruction leads to premature activation of pancreatic proenzymes (see above)

Inflammatory Cascade

▶ Recruitment and activation of complement system, neutrophils, and macrophages
▶ Release of proinflammatory cytokines into the systemic circulation
- For example, TNF-α, IL-1, IL-6

▶ Release of activated pancreatic enzymes into the systemic circulation

Systemic Response

▶ Circulating activated pancreatic enzymes and cytokines may lead to the systemic inflammatory response syndrome (see Chap. 15)
  • May lead to fever, ARDS, renal failure, and cardiovascular collapse
  • May also lead to loss of gastrointestinal integrity
    ○ May lead to bacterial translocation
      ▪ May lead to local or systemic infection
      ▪ Most infections in acute pancreatitis are caused by common enteric organisms
▶ Possible metabolic complications
  • Hypocalcemia
    ○ Usually secondary to calcium-soap formation
  • Hyperlipidemia
  • Hyperglycemia or hypoglycemia

Possible Etiologies

Gallstones

▶ Account for 35–45% of cases of acute pancreatitis
  • Most common cause
▶ Likely mechanisms
  • Obstruction at the ampulla of Vater
  • Reflux of bile into the pancreatic duct due to transient obstruction at the ampulla
▶ Usually caused by small stones with a diameter < 5 mm
  • Small enough to pass through the cystic duct and cause obstruction at the ampulla

Alcohol

▶ Accounts for 25–35% of cases of acute pancreatitis
  • Second most common cause
▶ Usually occurs in the setting of long-term alcohol abuse and not after an occasional binge
  • Often presents as an acute episode on a background of chronic pancreatitis
  • Signs of chronic pancreatitis include
    ○ Pancreatic calcification

- ○ Exocrine and/or endocrine dysfunction
- ○ Typical duct changes as seen on ERCP

Hypertriglyceridemia
- ▶ Usually need levels > 1000 mg/dl to precipitate acute pancreatitis
  - • Accounts for 1–4% of cases
- ▶ Pathogenesis of inflammation is unclear in this setting

Hypercalcemia
- ▶ Uncommon cause
- ▶ Usually caused by acute elevations as opposed to chronic elevations in serum calcium levels
  - • May involve deposition of calcium in the pancreatic duct and activation of trypsinogen

Medications
- ▶ May occur after a short duration, which is usually an immune-mediated allergic type reaction
- ▶ May occur after prolonged usage due to the accumulation of toxic metabolites
- ▶ Specific medications to consider
  - • Human immunodeficiency virus therapy
    - ○ Didanosine
    - ○ Pentamidine
  - • Antibiotics
    - ○ Metronidazole (Flagyl)
    - ○ Sulfonamides
    - ○ Tetracycline
  - • Diuretics
    - ○ Furosemide (Lasix)
    - ○ Thiazides
  - • Inflammatory bowel disease therapy
    - ○ Sulfasalazine
    - ○ 5-ASA
  - • Immunosuppressive agents
    - ○ Azathioprine
    - ○ L-Asparaginase
  - • Neuropsychiatric agents
    - ○ Valproic acid (Depakote)
  - • Antiinflammatory agents
    - ○ Sulindac
    - ○ Salicylates

- Miscellaneous
  - Calcium
  - Tamoxifen
  - Estrogen supplements

Infection
► Viruses
- Mumps
- Coxsackievirus
- Hepatitis B
- Cytomegalovirus
- Varicella-zoster
- Herpes simplex
- Human immunodeficiency virus (more commonly secondary to the medications used to treat the infection)
► Bacteria
- *Mycoplasma*
- *Legionella*
- *Leptospira*
- *Salmonella*
► Fungus
- *Aspergillus*
► Parasites
- *Toxoplasma*
- *Cryptosporidium*
- *Ascaris*

Trauma
► Uncommon cause
► May be secondary to blunt or penetrating injury
► Can range from mild contusion to complete transection of the gland

Pancreas Divisum
► Results from failure of the embryologically derived dorsal and ventral pancreas to fuse, which results in separate ductal systems
- Ventral: main duct of Wirsung
- Dorsal: accessory duct of Santorini
► Common anatomical variant
- Occurs in approximately 7% of autopsy series

▶ Controversial as to whether this is an etiology of acute pancreatitis
  • Ninety-five percent of patients diagnosed with pancreas divisum remain asymptomatic
  • Proposed mechanism of causing pancreatitis:
    ○ Narrow minor papilla through which the accessory duct of Santorini drains causes a relative obstruction to the flow of pancreatic secretions
      ▪ Leads to the premature activation of pancreatic proenzymes

Vascular Disease
▶ Ischemia is an uncommon cause.
▶ Consider the following causes:
  • Vasculitis
    ○ Systemic lupus erythematosus
    ○ Polyarteritis nodosa
  • Atheroembolism
  • Hypotension or shock

Pregnancy
▶ Rare cause of acute pancreatitis
▶ Most cases are related to pregnancy-related gallstones

Post–Endoscopic Retrograde Cholangiopancreatography
▶ Occurs in approximately 3–5% of patients undergoing diagnostic or therapeutic ERCP

Cystic Fibrosis
▶ Leads to "plugging" of the pancreatic duct
▶ Usually associated with chronic pancreatitis

Idiopathic
▶ Accounts for 20–30% of cases of acute pancreatitis
▶ Third most common cause (after gallstones and alcohol)

SYMPTOMS AND SIGNS

Symptoms
▶ Abdominal pain
  • Mid-epigastrium

- • Right upper quadrant
- • Diffuse
► Pain radiating to the back
► Nausea
► Vomiting
► Pain worse with eating and drinking

Signs

► Fever
► Tachycardia
► Tachypnea
► Abdominal examination
- • Tenderness
- • Guarding
- • Distention and decreased bowel sounds secondary to a functional ileus
► Ecchymotic discoloration (sign of hemorrhage)
- • Flank region (Grey-Turner's sign)
  - ○ Associated with retroperitoneal bleeding
- • Periumbilical region (Cullen's sign)
  - ○ Associated with intraperitoneal bleeding
► Mental status changes

DIAGNOSIS

General

► History
► Physical examination

Laboratory Tests

Serum Amylase
► Rises within 6–12 hours of onset of acute pancreatitis.
► Can be elevated in other conditions.
- • Mesenteric ischemia
  - ○ Increased transmural absorption
- • Perforated peptic ulcer
  - ○ Increased transperitoneal absorption

- Intestinal obstruction
  - Increased transmural absorption
- Biliary colic
  - May be secondary to subclinical underlying pancreatitis
- Renal failure
  - Reduced renal clearance of amylase
- Tubo-ovarian disease (ruptured ectopic pregnancy or salpingitis)
  - Secreted from fallopian tubes
- Excessive salivary gland production
- Macroamylasemia
  - Secondary to normal serum amylase being bound to abnormal serum proteins

▶ The degree of elevation does not reflect the severity of pancreatitis.

Serum Lipase

▶ Greater sensitivity and specificity than serum amylase levels.

▶ Enzyme levels tend to stay elevated longer than amylase levels.

- May be useful for patients who have delayed presentation from the onset of pancreatitis.

▶ The degree of elevation does not reflect the severity of pancreatitis.

Urine Amylase

▶ Amylase to creatinine clearance ratio increases from a normal 3% to approximately 10%.

- Renal insufficiency interferes with this test.

Liver Enzymes

▶ Elevated bilirubin (usually conjugated), transaminase enzymes (usually ALT), and alkaline phosphatase (least specific) suggest a gallstone etiology of the pancreatitis.

Radiographic Tests

Abdominal Plain Film

▶ Mostly helps to *exclude* other causes of acute abdominal pain such as obstruction and bowel perforation

► Localized ileus secondary to pancreatitis may be present on the film
  • "Sentinel loop"
    ○ Localized ileus of segment of small bowel
  • "Colon cutoff sign"
    ○ Paucity of air in the colon distal to the splenic flexure secondary to spasm of the colon in that area from the spread of pancreatic inflammation

Chest Radiograph
► Elevation of a hemidiaphragm
► Pleural effusions
► Basal atelectasis
► Presence of ARDS (see Chap. 19)

Right Upper Quadrant Ultrasound
► Assess for the presence of gallstones and/or biliary tree dilatation.
► Assess pancreatic head morphology.

Magnetic Resonance Cholangiopancreatography (MRCP)
► Useful imaging modality to assess the biliary tree if ultrasound is nondiagnostic
  • Assess for gallstones (either cholelithiasis or choledocholithiasis) and/or biliary tree dilatation.

Computerized Tomography
► Most valuable imaging tool for diagnosing *severe* pancreatitis
  • IV (renal function permitting) and oral contrast–enhanced scan should be obtained in patients suspected of having *severe* pancreatitis:
    ○ Can identify areas of pancreatic necrosis
    ○ Can identify other local complications such as abscess and pseudocyst (delayed complication)
  • Severity of pancreatitis can also be classified into five grades based on an *unenhanced* CT scan:
    ○ Grade A – normal pancreas consistent with mild pancreatitis
    ○ Grade B – focal or diffuse enlargement of the gland, but no peripancreatic inflammation

- ○ Grade C – abnormalities seen in grade B plus peripancreatic inflammation
- ○ Grade D – grade C plus associated single fluid collection
- ○ Grade E – grade C plus two or more peripancreatic fluid collections or gas in the pancreas or retroperitoneum

MANAGEMENT

Predicting Severity

- ▶ Scoring systems
  - Ranson criteria
    - ○ The presence of up to three of the following criteria represents mild pancreatitis, whereas the mortality rate rises significantly with four or more criteria:
      - ▪ At admission
        - ➢ Age > 55 years
        - ➢ White blood cell count > 16,000 cells/mm^3
        - ➢ Blood glucose > 200 mg/dl
        - ➢ Lactate dehydrogenase (LDH) > 350 IU/L
        - ➢ Aspartate transaminase (AST) > 250 IU/L
      - ▪ Forty-eight hours after admission
        - ➢ Hematocrit fall by ≥ 10%
        - ➢ BUN increase by 5 mg/dl
        - ➢ Serum calcium < 8 mg/dl
        - ➢ PaO_2 < 60 mmHg
        - ➢ Base deficit > 4 mmol/L
        - ➢ Fluid sequestration > 6 L
  - Acute physiology and chronic health evaluation (APACHE) II system
    - ○ Most commonly used scoring system for disease severity
    - ○ Can be used throughout the patient's hospitalization
- ▶ These systems provide a framework in which to stratify patients; however, should only be used as a *guide* to therapy, not to *direct* therapy.

Airway

- ▶ Ensure a stable airway.
  - Consider mechanical ventilation if necessary (see Chap. 4).

Oxygenation

▶ Optimize oxygenation (see Chap. 3).
   • Increase FIO_2.
   • Consider mechanical ventilation if necessary (see Chap. 4).

Supportive Management

▶ Nothing by mouth.
▶ If the patient is vomiting or has gastric dilatation secondary to an ileus, place a nasogastric tube for decompression.
▶ Provide adequate pain control (see Chap. 6).
▶ Correct or remove any reversible underlying suspected etiologies, such as hypercalcemia, hypertriglyceridemia, and medications.

Cardiovascular Support

▶ IV fluid resuscitation
   • Most patients require an aggressive fluid challenge.
   • Minimizes a pre-renal etiology of renal insufficiency.
   • Consider titrating fluid resuscitation to filling pressure measurements.
      ◦ Central venous catheter
         ▪ CVP 10–12 mmHg
      ◦ PA catheter (see Chap. 5)
         ▪ PCWP 18 mmHg
         ▪ Can also help guide vasopressor therapy
▶ Vasopressor therapy
   • Main goals
      ◦ Increase systemic vascular tone
      ◦ Optimize cardiac output and delivery of oxygen to peripheral tissues
   • Consider the following regimens (see Chap. 6)
      ◦ Norepinephrine (Levophed) ± vasopressin
         ▪ Consider as the first choice
         ▪ May add dopamine if the patient remains hypotensive on maximum doses of norepinephrine and vasopressin
      ◦ Dopamine ± vasopressin
         ▪ Use high doses of dopamine in order to target all receptors.
         ▪ Do *not* use "renal-dose dopamine."

    ◦   Dobutamine ± phenylephrine (Neo-Synephrine) ± vasopressin

Acute Respiratory Distress Syndrome

▶ If the patient develops ARDS
- Institute mechanical ventilation (see Chap. 4, Chap. 19).
- Consider specific ARDS therapeutic strategies (see Chap. 19).

Metabolic and Serum Glucose Abnormalities

▶ Correct metabolic/serum glucose abnormalities.
- Maintain serum glucose ≤ 120 mg/dl.

Renal Failure

▶ Consider instituting hemodialysis or continuous veno-venous hemofiltration (CVVH) in patients with renal failure unresponsive to IV fluid therapy or severe metabolic derangements.

Antimicrobial Therapy

▶ Indications
- Suspected biliary sepsis
  - ◦ Usually from an obstructing gallstone
- Suspected infectious etiology of pancreatitis
- Presence of pancreatic necrosis
  - ◦ Administer imipenem (Primaxin)
    - ▪ Dose: 250–1000 mg IV q 6–8 hours
    - ▪ Duration: 7–14 days
- Presence of infection at another site
  - ◦ Urinary tract infection
  - ◦ Pneumonia
  - ◦ Blood
    - ▪ Catheter-related infection

Nutrition

▶ See Chap. 9.
▶ Enteral route
- Advantages
  - ◦ Avoids catheter-related infections.

- o Maintains gut barrier integrity.
- o Theoretically reduces risk of bacterial translocation.
- o Studies have shown that early enteral feeding significantly decreases systemic inflammatory response syndrome and the incidence of septic complications.
- Can be delivered using a nasojejunal (post-ligament of Treitz) feeding tube
  - o Avoids the concern of pancreatic stimulation with gastric feeding
  - o Does not worsen pancreatitis as determined by CT scan scores
- ▶ Parenteral route
  - Administer parenteral nutrition if there is a contraindication to enteral feeding, such as a severe intestinal ileus.

Specific Management of Pancreatic Necrosis

- ▶ Administer empiric antibiotic therapy using imipenem.
- ▶ Difficult to distinguish sterile from infected pancreatic necrosis.
  - Infection, when present, usually occurs during the second to third week of the clinical course.
    - o Often associated with air seen in the pancreatic bed on CT scan.
  - Must eliminate all other sources of possible infection.
  - If infected pancreatic necrosis is still suspected:
    - o May proceed with a CT-guided percutaneous aspiration of necrotic tissue.
      - ▪ Send the aspirate for Gram stain and culture.
        - ➤ If the aspirate is sterile, continue with medical management.
    - o May proceed directly to surgical débridement if the patient is hemodynamically unstable.
  - If infected pancreatic necrosis is documented:
    - o Proceed with surgical debridement of infected tissue.

Specific Management of Gallstone Pancreatitis

- ▶ For *severe* pancreatitis, consider early ERCP (within 48 hours of clinical course) to provide endoscopic biliary and pancreatic duct decompression.

- ▶ Cholecystectomy should be performed after pancreatitis has resolved and the patient is stable.
  - Most prefer to do this *before* the patient's discharge from the hospital.
- ▶ Should document adequate drainage of the biliary tree.
  - Preoperative ERCP
  - Cholecystectomy with intraoperative cholangiogram
  - Postoperative ERCP
  - Magnetic resonance cholangiopancreatography

Additional Treatments

- ▶ Administer DVT prophylaxis (see Chap. 10).
- ▶ Administer stress ulcer prophylaxis (see Chap. 10).

CHAPTER 17

FULMINANT HEPATIC FAILURE

ABBREVIATIONS

ARDS: acute respiratory distress syndrome
ATPase: adenosine triphosphatase
CVP: central venous pressure
FDA: U.S. Food and Drug Administration
FFP: fresh frozen plasma
FIO_2: inspired fraction of oxygen
HELLP: hemolysis, elevated liver-enzyme levels, low platelets
ICP: intracranial pressure
INR: international normalized ratio
NAPQI: N-acetyl-p-benzoquinoneimine
NO: nitric oxide
PA: pulmonary artery
PCWP: pulmonary capillary wedge pressure
PEEP: positive end-expiratory pressure
PT: prothrombin time
PTT: partial thromboplastin time

DEFINITION

► Hyperacute liver failure
  • Onset of hepatic encephalopathy within 7 days of jaundice
► Acute liver failure
  • Onset of hepatic encephalopathy within 8–28 days of jaundice
► Subacute liver failure
  • Onset of hepatic encephalopathy within 5–12 weeks of jaundice

▶ Hepatic encephalopathy
- A reversible syndrome of impaired brain function that occurs in patients with advanced liver failure
- Grading system
  ○ Grade I
    - Mild confusion
    - Decreased attention
    - Irritability
    - Disordered sleep
  ○ Grade II
    - Intermittent disorientation
    - Moderate confusion
    - Drowsiness/lethargy
    - Personality changes
  ○ Grade III
    - Gross disorientation
    - Marked confusion
    - Incoherent
    - Sleeping but arousable
  ○ Grade IV
    - Frank coma

PATHOPHYSIOLOGY

Effect on Organ Systems

Liver failure can affect and compromise all organ systems.

Central Nervous System
▶ Hepatic encephalopathy
- Increased NH_3 levels (currently believed to be the main etiology)
  ○ The gastrointestinal tract is the primary source of NH_3.
    - Produced by enterocytes from glutamine
    - Produced by colonic bacterial catabolism of nitrogenous substances such as protein
  ○ An intact liver clears almost all of the NH_3 that enters the portal circulation from the gastrointestinal tract.

- Liver failure leads to increased systemic circulating NH_3 levels.
  - Increases the cerebral uptake of neutral amino acids
    - May affect the synthesis of neurotransmitters such as dopamine, norepinephrine, and serotonin
    - Leads to encephalopathy
- Increased ratio of plasma aromatic amino acids to branched-chain amino acids (suggested as a second or adjunct etiology)
  - May lead to increased brain levels of aromatic amino acid precursors for neurotransmitters and lead to altered neuronal excitability
- ► Increased cerebral edema
  - Develops in 75–80% of patients with grade IV encephalopathy
  - Possible etiologies
    - Vasogenic edema secondary to increased blood–brain barrier permeability
    - Direct cytotoxicity from the osmotic effects of NH_3, glutamine, and other amino acids
    - Dysfunction of the sodium-potassium ATPase pump
  - Can lead to elevated ICP (see Chap. 7)
    - Can lead to brainstem herniation, which is the most common cause of death from fulminant hepatic failure
    - Can also lead to ischemic and hypoxic injury to the brain due to reduced cerebral perfusion pressure (see Chap. 7)

Cardiovascular
- ► Can lead to systemic vasodilatation
  - May be secondary to increased NO levels
  - Specific alterations that may occur (resembles septic shock, see Chap. 5, Chap. 15)
    - Hypotension
    - Decreased systemic vascular resistance
    - Compensatory increase in cardiac output
- ► Increased interstitial edema

Pulmonary
- ► Increased risk of pulmonary edema
- ► Increased risk of pneumonia
  - Attenuated immune system
  - Encephalopathy can increase the risk of aspiration

▶ May lead to ARDS (see Chap. 19)

Gastrointestinal
▶ Increased risk of developing stress ulcers
▶ May lead to diffuse ileus

Renal
▶ May lead to acute renal failure
  • Must first exclude the usual pre-renal, renal, and post-renal causes of acute renal failure
    ◦ Pre-renal
      ▪ Usually secondary to hypovolemia
    ◦ Renal
      ▪ Acute tubular necrosis
        ➢ Toxin induced
          ❖ May be the same toxin that led to liver failure (e.g., acetaminophen)
        ➢ Ischemia induced
      ▪ Acute interstitial nephritis
        ➢ Usually toxin induced
      ▪ Glomerulonephritis
    ◦ Post-renal
      ▪ Usually secondary to obstruction
  • Consider the hepatorenal syndrome
    ◦ Diagnosis of exclusion
      ▪ Associated with the following parameters:
        ➢ Urine volume < 500 ml/day
        ➢ Urine sodium < 10 mEq/L
        ➢ Urine osmolarity greater than the plasma osmolarity
        ➢ Urine blood cells < 50/high-power field
        ➢ Serum sodium concentration < 130 mEq/L
    ◦ May be precipitated by an infection from another source (e.g., spontaneous bacterial peritonitis)
    ◦ Thought to be caused by increased splanchnic vasodilatation
      ▪ Leads to decreased renal blood flow, glomerular filtration rate, and creatinine clearance

Immune System
▶ Increased risk of infection:
  • Complement deficiency
  • Reduced opsonization
  • White blood cell dysfunction
  • Altered killer cell function
▶ Sepsis is the second most common cause of death from fulminant hepatic failure.

Hematologic
▶ Platelets
  • Decreased platelet count
  • Altered platelet function
▶ Coagulation factors
  • Decreased hepatic synthesis of clotting factors
    ○ Leads to increased PT/PTT/INR
▶ Increased risk of bleeding

Metabolic
▶ Decreased hepatic gluconeogenesis
  • May lead to hypoglycemia
▶ Possible electrolyte abnormalities
  • Hypokalemia
  • Hyponatremia
  • Hypophosphatemia

Possible Etiologies

Viral
▶ Hepatitis A
  • Rare cause of fulminant hepatic failure
▶ Hepatitis B
  • Most common viral cause
▶ Hepatitis C
  • Not a major cause of fulminant hepatic failure
▶ Other viruses to consider
  • Hepatitis D
    ○ Usually as a coinfection

- Hepatitis E
  - More common in pregnancy in endemic areas
- Epstein-Barr virus
- Cytomegalovirus
- Herpes simplex virus
- Varicella-zoster

Toxic
► Acetaminophen (paracetamol)
  - Most common toxin:
    - Usually associated with a suicide attempt
  - Toxic dose:
    - Child: 150 mg/kg
    - Adult: 7.5–10 g/day
  - Toxicity is secondary to accumulation of toxic metabolite NAPQI.
    - Toxic doses of acetaminophen saturate the normal glucuronide metabolic pathway, which leads to increased production of NAPQI through the cytochrome P-450 metabolic pathway.
    - Normally, hepatic glutathione rapidly conjugates NAPQI, which then leads to renal excretion.
    - Toxic doses deplete hepatic glutathione stores.
      - Chronic alcohol ingestion also depletes glutathione stores and upregulates cytochrome P-450 activity.
        - Can increase the susceptibility to acetaminophen toxicity.
    - Accumulation of NAPQI leads to oxidative injury and hepatocellular necrosis.
► Other potential toxins to consider
  - Isoniazid
  - Valproate
  - Halothane
  - Phenytoin
  - Sulfonamides
  - Propylthiouracil
  - Amiodarone
  - Disulfiram
  - Dapsone
  - Mushrooms

Vascular
► Hepatic ischemia
    • May be secondary to myocardial infarction, cardiomyopathy, or pulmonary embolism
► Hepatic venous outflow occlusion
    • Hepatic vein thrombosis (Budd-Chiari syndrome)
    • Veno-occlusive disease
► Portal vein thrombosis

Metabolic
► Wilson disease
► Acute fatty liver of pregnancy
    • Usually occurs in the third trimester
► HELLP syndrome
► Reye's syndrome

Miscellaneous
► Malignant infiltration of the liver
► Sepsis
► Heat stroke
► Autoimmune hepatitis

SYMPTOMS AND SIGNS

Symptoms
► Nonspecific
► Abdominal pain
► Altered mental status
► Malaise
► Nausea/vomiting
► Dyspnea

Signs
► Fever
► Tachycardia
► Tachypnea
► Hypotension
► Oliguria
► Confusion

▶ Jaundice
▶ Evidence of bleeding

DIAGNOSIS

General

▶ History
▶ Physical examination
▶ Altered mental status

Laboratory Tests

▶ Prolonged PT (increased INR)
▶ Elevated liver enzyme levels
▶ Thrombocytopenia
▶ Electrolyte abnormalities
▶ Hypoglycemia
▶ Viral serology
▶ Toxicology screen
  • Elevated acetaminophen levels
  • Elevated serum levels of other possible toxins
▶ Blood cultures
  • Assess for septicemia

Radiographic Tests

▶ Usually not needed to make the diagnosis
▶ May be useful in excluding other possible etiologies of the patient's clinical status or to recognize the less common causes of fulminant hepatic failure

Ultrasound

▶ Can assess blood flow in the hepatic artery, hepatic vein, and portal vein

Computerized Tomography Scan (Contrast Enhanced)

▶ Can assess blood flow in the hepatic artery, hepatic vein, and portal vein
▶ Can assess for malignant infiltration of the liver

MANAGEMENT

Central Nervous System

▶ Hepatic encephalopathy
- Ensure a stable airway.
  ○ Consider mechanical ventilation if necessary (see Chap. 4).
- Lactulose:
  ○ Mechanisms of action
    ▪ Lowers colonic pH, which favors the formation of nonabsorbable NH_4^+ from NH_3.
      ➢ Retains NH_3 in the colon.
      ➢ Reduces plasma NH_3 concentrations.
    ▪ Has a cathartic effect, which improves a functional ileus.
    ▪ Increases fecal nitrogen excretion secondary to the increased stool volume.
  ○ Dose
    ▪ 45–90 g PO QD divided TID/QID.
    ▪ May also be given as an enema.
    ▪ Titrate dose to two to four soft stools per day.
- Dietary protein reduction:
  ○ Maintain daily protein intake between 40 and 70 g/day.
  ○ Avoid large negative nitrogen balance (see Chap. 9).
  ○ Administering branched-chain amino acids has *not* been shown to be of therapeutic benefit.
- Oral neomycin:
  ○ Mechanism of action:
    ▪ Inhibits NH_3 production by eradicating NH_3-producing bacteria.
  ○ Dose:
    ▪ 2–8 g PO/NG QD divided QID.
    ▪ Monitor for ototoxicity and nephrotoxicity.
  ○ Usually reserved for patients *not* responding to lactulose and protein reduction therapy.
▶ Increased cerebral edema
- Consider invasive ICP monitoring for patients with grade III/IV encephalopathy (see Chap. 7)
- Follow elevated ICP management protocol (see Chap. 7)

Cardiovascular

▶ IV fluid resuscitation
- Most patients require an aggressive fluid challenge.
  - ○ Crystalloid and colloid therapy (see Chap. 6).
  - ○ Monitor for worsening cerebral edema.
- Consider titrating fluid resuscitation to filling pressure measurements.
  - ○ Central venous catheter
    - ▪ CVP 10–12 mmHg
  - ○ PA catheter (see Chap. 5)
    - ▪ PCWP 18 mmHg
  - ○ Can also help guide vasopressor therapy
▶ Vasopressor therapy
- Main goals:
  - ○ Increase systemic vascular tone
  - ○ Optimize cardiac output and delivery of oxygen to peripheral tissues (see Chap. 3)
- Consider the following regimens (see Chap. 6):
  - ○ Norepinephrine (Levophed) ± vasopressin
    - ▪ Consider as the first choice
    - ▪ May add dopamine if the patient remains hypotensive on maximum doses of norepinephrine and vasopressin
  - ○ Dopamine ± vasopressin
    - ▪ Use high doses of dopamine to target all receptors.
    - ▪ Do *not* use "renal-dose dopamine."
  - ○ Dobutamine ± phenylephrine (Neo-Synephrine) ± vasopressin

Pulmonary

▶ Ensure a secure airway.
▶ Optimize oxygenation (see Chap. 3, Chap. 4).
- Increase FIO_2.
- If mechanically ventilated, consider administering PEEP (see Chap. 4).
  - ○ Monitor for increasing ICP with administration of PEEP due to the possibility of reduced cerebral venous drainage.
▶ If the patient develops ARDS:
- Institute mechanical ventilation (see Chap. 4, Chap. 19).
- Consider specific ARDS therapeutic strategies (see Chap. 19).

Gastrointestinal

▶ Administer stress ulcer prophylaxis (see Chap. 10).

Renal

▶ Pre-renal, renal, or post-renal causes
  • Treat the underlying etiology
    ○ Ensure euvolemia
    ○ Remove potential toxins
    ○ Remove obstruction
▶ Hepatorenal syndrome
  • Midodrine (ProAmatine)
    ○ Selective α_1-receptor agonist
      ▪ Applies vasoconstriction
    ○ Dose
      ▪ 5.0–12.5 mg PO/NG TID
  • Octreotide (Sandostatin)
    ○ Somatostatin analog
      ▪ Inhibitor of endogenous vasodilator release
    ○ Dose
      ▪ 100–200 µg SC TID
▶ Consider instituting hemodialysis or continuous venovenous hemofiltration/continuous venovenous hemodialysis in patients with renal failure unresponsive to the above therapies or severe metabolic derangements

Immune System

▶ Maintain a low threshold for obtaining cultures (blood, urine, sputum, ascites).
▶ Administer empiric broad-spectrum antibiotics while awaiting culture results (see Chap. 15).
▶ Administer empiric antifungal coverage if fungal infection is suspected (see Chap. 15).

Hematologic (Coagulopathy)

▶ Platelets (see Chap. 6)
  • Keep above 10,000–20,000.
  • Transfuse to > 50,000 before invasive procedures.

▶ FFP (see Chap. 6)
  • Prophylactic transfusion for elevated INR has *not* been shown to be beneficial.
  • Should be administered in the setting of active bleeding.
    ◦ Most common site of bleeding is the gastrointestinal tract

Metabolic

▶ Correct hypoglycemia.
▶ Correct electrolyte abnormalities.

Nutrition

▶ Administer early nutrition (see Chap. 9).
▶ Use the parenteral route if enteral feeding is not possible.
▶ Daily protein intake should be between 40 and 70 g/day.
▶ Branched-chain amino acids have *not* been shown to be beneficial.

Liver Transplantation

▶ Patients with fulminant hepatic failure should be managed in a liver transplant center.
▶ King's College Hospital criteria for liver transplantation:
  • Acetaminophen-induced disease
    ◦ Arterial pH < 7.3, or
    ◦ Grade III/IV encephalopathy and PT > 100 seconds and serum creatinine > 3.4 mg/dl
  • All other causes of fulminant hepatic failure
    ◦ PT > 100 seconds, or
    ◦ Any three of the following:
      ▪ Age < 10 years or > 40 years
      ▪ Etiology: non-A, non-B hepatitis, halothane hepatitis, idiosyncratic drug reaction
      ▪ Duration of jaundice before onset of encephalopathy > 7 days
      ▪ PT > 50 seconds
      ▪ Serum bilirubin > 18 mg/dl

Management Considerations for Specific Etiologies

Acetaminophen Toxicity
► Activated charcoal
  • Indicated for patients who present within 4 hours of inges-
    tion to provide gastrointestinal decontamination
  • Dose
    ○ 25–100 g PO/NG as a single dose
    ○ If multiple doses are needed, may administer 12.5 g PO/
      NG q hour as needed
► N-acetylcysteine
  • Mechanism of action
    ○ Repletes glutathione stores and thus limits the formation
      and accumulation of NAPQI
    ○ Combines directly with NAPQI as a glutathione
      substitute
    ○ Has antiinflammatory and antioxidant effects
    ○ Has inotropic and vasodilating effects
      ▪ May improve systemic oxygen delivery
  • Most effective when initiated within 10 hours of ingestion
  • Dose
    ○ Oral
      ▪ 72-hour course
      ▪ Loading dose: 140 mg/kg PO/NG once
      ▪ Maintenance dose: 70 mg/kg PO/NG q 4 hours
        times 17 doses
      ▪ Total dose: 1330 mg/kg
    ○ IV (recently FDA approved)
      ▪ 20-hour course
      ▪ Loading dose: 150 mg/kg IV once over 15 minutes
      ▪ Maintenance dose
        ➢ 50 mg/kg IV infusion over first 4 hours
        ➢ 100 mg/kg IV infusion over next 16 hours

Acute Budd-Chiari Syndrome
► Transjugular intrahepatic portosystemic shunt (TIPS)
► Surgical decompression
► Thrombolysis

Herpes Simplex Virus Infection
- ▶ Acyclovir (Zovirax)
  - • Dose: 5–10 mg/kg IV q 8 hours

Acute Fatty Liver of Pregnancy or HELLP Syndrome
- ▶ Consider delivery of fetus.

CHAPTER 18

VENOUS THROMBOEMBOLISM

ABBREVIATIONS

BP: blood pressure
CVP: central venous pressure
CXR: chest x-ray
DVT: deep venous thrombosis
FIO_2: inspired fraction of oxygen
HIT: heparin-induced thrombocytopenia
INR: international normalized ratio
IVC: inferior vena cava
LV: left ventricular
PA: pulmonary artery
$PaCO_2$: partial pressure of carbon dioxide (mmHg) – arterial
PaO_2: partial pressure of oxygen (mmHg) – arterial
PCWP: pulmonary capillary wedge pressure
PE: pulmonary embolism
PIOPED: Prospective Investigation of Pulmonary Embolus Diagnosis
PTT: partial thromboplastin time
RV: right ventricular
V/Q: ventilation/perfusion

DEFINITION

▶ Proximal DVT of the lower extremities
  • Located within the popliteal, femoral (including the superficial femoral), and iliac veins
    ○ Source of > 70% of all pulmonary emboli
    ○ Superior vena cava, upper extremity veins, gonadal veins, and right chambers of the heart are less common sources of PE

▶ Pulmonary embolism (PE)
  • Occurs when a segment of thrombus detaches from the vessel and travels to the lungs to lodge with the pulmonary arterial system

PATHOPHYSIOLOGY

Deep Venous Thrombosis

▶ Risk factors
  • Virchow's triad
    ○ Endothelial injury
    ○ Stasis of blood flow
    ○ Hypercoagulable state
      ▪ Specific hypercoagulable states to consider
        ➢ Factor V Leiden (most common)
        ➢ Presence of antiphospholipid antibodies
          ❖ Presence of anticardiolipin antibody
          ❖ Presence of lupus anticoagulant
        ➢ Hyperhomocysteinemia (accompanied by homocysteinuria)
        ➢ Protein C deficiency
        ➢ Protein S deficiency
        ➢ Antithrombin III deficiency
        ➢ Malignancy
▶ Involves accumulation of platelets and fibrin to form a thrombus
  • Endogenous fibrinolysis results in partial or complete resolution of the thrombus.
  • Residual thrombus becomes organized:
    ○ May incompletely recanalize, which may result in
      ▪ Narrowing of the vessel lumen
      ▪ Valvular incompetence
      ▪ Development of a collateral network
▶ Potential local complications
  • Infection of the thrombus (thrombophlebitis)
    ○ May lead to bacteremia or septicemia
  • Phlegmasia alba dolens
    ○ Large, swollen, and painful limb made pale by severe edema.
    ○ Associated lymphangitis is often present.
  • Phlegmasia cerulea dolens
    ○ Large, swollen, and painful leg that appears blue because of impending venous infarction

Pulmonary Embolism

▶ Thrombi usually lodge in lobar arteries or the distal main pulmonary artery.
   • Larger thrombi can also form a saddle embolus, which straddles the pulmonary artery bifurcation.
   • Smaller thrombi can travel to more distal, smaller arteries.
▶ Possible physiologic changes:
   • Increased dead space (see Chap. 3)
      ○ Leads to alveolar hyperventilation
   • Development of intrapulmonary shunt (see Chap. 3)
      ○ Leads to hypoxia
   • Development of atelectasis and edema
      ○ Usually secondary to decreased alveolar surfactant
   • Increased pulmonary vascular resistance
      ○ May lead to the acute development of pulmonary hypertension
         ▪ May lead to right ventricular failure
            ➤ May cause LV failure, a decrease in cardiac output, and hemodynamic instability
               ❖ RV failure can lead to the intraventricular septum bulging into the LV, thus causing LV diastolic dysfunction (see Chap. 1).
               ❖ LV diastolic dysfunction can lead to decreased cardiac output and hypotension.
               ❖ Hypotension, coupled with increased LV wall tension, can compromise coronary perfusion to the LV myocardium, thus leading to systolic dysfunction.

SYMPTOMS AND SIGNS

Symptoms

▶ DVT
   • Leg pain
   • Edema
   • Erythema
   • Warmth
   • May be asymptomatic
▶ PE
   • Dyspnea
   • Pleuritic chest pain

- Cough
- Hemoptysis
- Palpitations
- May be asymptomatic

Signs

▶ DVT
  - Leg edema
  - Erythema
  - Warmth
  - Distention of collateral veins
    ○ Not a common finding
  - Homan's sign
    ○ Calf pain with dorsiflexion of the foot
    ○ Insensitive and nonspecific sign
  - Lowenberg's sign
    ○ Calf pain with low pressure inflation of a blood pressure cuff
    ○ Insensitive and nonspecific sign
  - Palpable cord if there is an associated superficial vein thrombosis
  - May have no associated physical findings
▶ PE
  - Tachycardia
  - Tachypnea
  - Rales
  - Exaggerated second heart sound (S_2)
  - Presence of a fourth heart sound (S_4)
  - Diaphoresis
  - May have no associated physical findings

DIAGNOSIS

Deep Venous Thrombosis

General
▶ History
▶ Physical examination

Duplex Ultrasonography
► Combines B-mode imaging and Doppler techniques
► Most commonly used test
► > 95% sensitivity and specificity for proximal DVT
  • Less diagnostic for calf vein thrombosis
► Noninvasive
► Cannot always distinguish between an acute and chronic thrombus

D-Dimers
► Formed when plasmin degrades cross-linked fibrin
► Nonsensitive, but a very specific test
  • Most useful for *excluding* DVT rather than making the diagnosis.
  • A D-dimer level of < 500 ng/ml has a negative predictive value of 95%.
► Can be elevated in other conditions
  • Recent surgery
  • Recent trauma
  • Infection
  • Active cardiopulmonary disease
  • Renal insufficiency
  • Malignancy
  • Disseminated intravascular coagulation (DIC)

Contrast Venography
► Gold standard
► Rarely used
  • Invasive
    ○ Requires placement of a tourniquet to occlude the superficial veins.
    ○ Contrast is injected into a superficial vein on the dorsum of the patient's foot.
    ○ Contrast travels through the perforating veins to reach the deep system, because the superficial veins have been occluded with a tourniquet.
  • Exposes the patient to IV contrast

Impedance Plethysmography
▶ Uses electrodes placed around the calf to measure changes in blood volume
  • A proximal DVT (obstruction) usually increases the blood volume in the calf.
  • Increased blood volume decreases electrical impedance.
▶ Very sensitive and specific test for making the diagnosis
▶ Rarely used since duplex ultrasonography has become widely available

Magnetic Resonance Venography
▶ Similar sensitivity and specificity as contrast venography
▶ Rarely used to make the diagnosis
  • High cost
  • Patient discomfort

Pulmonary Embolism

General
▶ History
▶ Physical examination

Electrocardiogram
▶ May be normal
▶ Sinus tachycardia
  • Most common finding
▶ Evidence of right heart strain
  • Right axis deviation
  • Right bundle branch block
  • P-wave pulmonale
  • $S_1Q_3T_3$ pattern
    ○ Prominent S waves in lead I
    ○ Q waves in lead III
    ○ T-wave inversion in lead III
▶ Nonspecific ST–T wave changes
  • T-wave inversion in leads V_1–V_4
▶ Dysrhythmias

Arterial Blood Gas
▶ May be normal
▶ Normal or low $PaCO_2$
  • Secondary to hyperventilation

▶ Low PaO$_2$
  • Secondary to intrapulmonary shunt
  • Increased alveolar-arterial oxygen gradient (see Chap. 3)

Chest Radiograph
▶ May be normal
▶ Nonspecific changes
  • Pleural effusions
  • Atelectasis
  • Elevation of a hemidiaphragm
  • Infiltrates
▶ Classic signs (only occasionally seen)
  • Hampton hump
    ○ Wedge-shaped opacity along the pleural surface
  • Westermark sign
    ○ Wedge-shaped loss of vascularity
  • Palla sign
    ○ Enlarged right descending pulmonary artery

Lung Scintigraphy (Ventilation/Perfusion Scan)
▶ Detects areas of "mismatch" between ventilation and perfusion
▶ Need a baseline CXR to properly interpret a V/Q scan
  • Other conditions can cause defects in ventilation and/or perfusion
    ○ Postoperative atelectasis
    ○ Pulmonary edema
    ○ Pulmonary infiltrate
    ○ Previous PE
    ○ Interstitial fibrosis
▶ Diagnostic accuracy is highly associated with pretest clinical suspicion of PE (PIOPED study; Table 18-1)

TABLE 18-1.
PROBABILITY OF PULMONARY EMBOLISM

V/Q scan probability	Clinical probability		
	High (%)	Intermediate (%)	Low (%)
High	96	88	56
Intermediate	66	28	16
Low	40	16	4

Spiral (Helical) Computerized Tomography
- ▶ Enables visualization of intraluminal filling defect in pulmonary arterial system
  - • More sensitive for emboli in main, lobar, and segmental pulmonary arteries compared to more peripheral areas
- ▶ Widely used diagnostic test
- ▶ Exposes the patient to IV contrast
  - • Must be cautious in patients with renal insufficiency

Echocardiography
- ▶ Used to assess for right ventricular dysfunction
- ▶ Transthoracic and/or transesophageal techniques can be used

Pulmonary Angiography
- ▶ Gold standard
- ▶ Rarely used
  - • Invasive
  - • Exposes the patient to IV contrast
  - • High cost

MANAGEMENT

Airway

- ▶ Ensure a stable airway.
  - • Consider mechanical ventilation if necessary (see Chap. 4).

Oxygenation

- ▶ Optimize oxygenation (see Chap. 3).
  - • Increase FIO_2.
  - • Consider mechanical ventilation if necessary (see Chap. 4).

Heparin

- ▶ See Chap. 10.
- ▶ Recommended weight-based dosing (often *overestimates* dose):
  - • Loading dose: 80 U/kg IV bolus (maximum, 5000 U).
  - • Infusion: 18 U/kg/hr.
  - • Titrate dose to a PTT value of 1.5–2.5 times normal value.

- Check PTT 6 hours after altering infusion rate.
  - ○ Half-life of heparin is 90 minutes and steady state is reached after 4 half-lives.
▶ Be cautious of potential complications.
- Bleeding
- HIT-I/HIT-II (see Chap. 10)

Low-Molecular-Weight Heparin

▶ See Chap. 10.
▶ Similar efficacy as standard heparin therapy.
- May have a lower risk of bleeding.
- Lower risk of developing HIT-I/HIT-II.
- Not reversible and dose is not easily titratable.
  - ○ Be cautious when administering to patients with renal insufficiency because its primary route of clearance is renal.
▶ Recommended weight-based dosing:
- Enoxaparin (Lovenox): 1 mg/kg SC BID.
- Tinzaparin (Innohep): 175 U/kg SC QD.
- Laboratory monitoring of dosage is usually *not* necessary due to a predictable dose–response relationship.
  - ○ Can measure activated factor X levels

Note: Dalteparin (Fragmin) is approved by the U.S. Food and Drug Administration only for *prophylaxis* of DVT.

Warfarin (Coumadin)

▶ Inhibits gamma-carboxylation of the vitamin-K–dependent clotting factors II, VII, IX, X, protein C, protein S.
▶ Recommended dosing:
- Usual dose: 2–5 mg PO QD.
  - ○ May consider using higher doses (5–10 mg) to provide a "loading" dose for the first 2–3 days of initiating therapy.
    - ▪ Can result in excessive anticoagulation and potential bleeding complications.
  - ○ Metabolized by cytochrome P-450 enzymes in the liver.
    - ▪ May be affected by other medications that alter cytochrome P-450 function.
- Titrate dose to a target INR of 2.0–3.0.
  - ○ Dose can be affected by patient factors.
    - ▪ Poor nutritional status.
      - ➢ Consider decreasing warfarin dose.

- Concurrent antibiotic therapy.
  - ➤ Can reduce colonic bacterial flora that produce vitamin K.
  - ➤ Consider decreasing warfarin dose.
- Mechanical bowel preparation.
  - ➤ Can reduce colonic bacterial flora that produce vitamin K.
  - ➤ Consider decreasing warfarin dose.
▶ Concomitant administration of heparin/low-molecular-weight heparin should be used for the first 3 days to avoid the theoretical risk of hypercoagulability associated with initiating warfarin therapy.
  - Hypercoagulability is secondary to the inhibition of protein C and protein S, which have the shortest half-lives of all the vitamin-K–dependent clotting factors.

Duration of Anticoagulation Therapy

▶ Should be individualized for each patient
  - Age
  - Comorbidities
  - Presence of hypercoagulable states
  - Reversible etiology of thromboembolism (surgery, trauma, immobilization, estrogen use)
▶ Range: 3 months to lifetime
  - Six months is preferable to 3 months

Inferior Vena Cava Filter

▶ Used to prevent pulmonary embolization of a thrombus
▶ Indications
  - Patients at high risk for venous thromboembolism in whom anticoagulation therapy is contraindicated (e.g., patients with closed head injury)
  - Patients who have recurrent thromboembolism despite adequate anticoagulation
▶ Placement
  - Should be placed in an *infra-renal* position.
    - ○ Avoids renal failure in the case of IVC thrombosis secondary to the filter being in place.

- Temporary IVC filters can be placed which can be retrieved at a later date.
  - The length of time of retrievability is variable depending on the type of filter.
- Placement of an IVC filter does *not* preclude anticoagulation therapy in those patients whom are eligible.
  - Anticoagulation can prevent the development of local complications secondary to the DVT.

Cardiovascular Support for the Hemodynamically Unstable Patient

▶ IV fluid resuscitation
- Most patients require a fluid challenge.
- Consider titrating fluid resuscitation to filling pressure measurements.
  - Central venous catheter
    - CVP 10–12 mmHg
  - PA catheter (see Chap. 5)
    - PCWP 18 mmHg
  - Can also help guide vasopressor therapy

Vasopressor Therapy

▶ Main goals:
- Increase systemic vascular tone.
  - Increases diastolic BP, which can improve coronary perfusion to the myocardium.
- Optimize cardiac output and delivery of oxygen to peripheral tissues (See Chap. 3).
  - Medications with β_2 agonist properties can also decrease the pulmonary vascular resistance.
▶ Consider the following regimens (see Chap. 6):
- Norepinephrine (Levophed) ± vasopressin
  - Consider as the first choice.
  - May add dopamine if the patient remains hypotensive on maximum doses of norepinephrine and vasopressin.
- Dopamine ± vasopressin
  - Use high doses of dopamine in order to target all receptors.
  - Do *not* use "renal-dose dopamine."
- Dobutamine ± phenylephrine (Neo-Synephrine) ± vasopressin

Thrombolytic Therapy

▶ Potential indications:
- Massive iliofemoral thrombus
- Presence of phlegmasia cerulea dolens
- Hemodynamic instability

▶ Medications:
- Alteplase (t-PA, Activase)
  ○ Dose: 100 mg IV over 2 hours
- Streptokinase (Streptase)
  ○ Loading dose: 250,000 IU IV bolus over 30 minutes
  ○ Infusion: 100,000 IU/hr IV
    ▪ PE: continue infusion for 24 hours.
    ▪ DVT: continue infusion for up to 72 hours.

▶ Be cautious of possible bleeding complications.

Inhaled Nitric Oxide

▶ Mechanism of action
- Causes vasodilatation of the pulmonary arterial system
- Reduces pulmonary hypertension
- May improve right ventricular function
- May lead to systemic hemodynamic improvement

▶ Dose
- No dose-response curves have been established.
- Consider starting with 5 parts per million (ppm) and titrate to effect.

▶ May be used as an adjunctive therapy in hemodynamically unstable patients along with vasopressors, thrombolytics, and/or embolectomy

Pulmonary Embolectomy

▶ Consider for patients with hemodynamic instability refractory to vasopressor therapy and have either failed, or have a contra-indication to, thrombolytic therapy.

▶ Rarely performed.

▶ Performed using a percutaneous interventional or an open surgical technique.

▶ High mortality rate.

CHAPTER 19

ACUTE RESPIRATORY DISTRESS SYNDROME

ABBREVIATIONS

ABG: arterial blood gas
ARDS: acute respiratory distress syndrome
CHF: congestive heart failure
CXR: chest x-ray
CO: cardiac output
DO_2: delivery of oxygen (ml O_2/min)
FIO_2: inspired fraction of oxygen
FRC: functional residual capacity
ICP: intracranial pressure
IL: interleukin
Map: mean airway pressure
MV: minute ventilation
$PaCO_2$: partial pressure of carbon dioxide (mmHg) – arterial
PaO_2: partial pressure of oxygen (mmHg) – arterial
PAWP: pulmonary artery wedge pressure
PEEP: positive end-expiratory pressure
TNF-α: tumor necrosis factor alpha
V/Q: ventilation/perfusion
Vt: tidal volume

DEFINITION

► Acute onset
► Bilateral diffuse alveolar infiltrates
► PAWP ≤ 18 mmHg
► Acute lung injury
  • PaO_2:FIO_2 ratio ≤ 300
► ARDS
  • PaO_2:FIO_2 ratio ≤ 200

PATHOPHYSIOLOGY

Caused by a Network of Cytokines

▶ For example, IL-1, IL-6, IL-8, IL-10, TNF-α.
▶ Cytokines initiate and amplify the lung injury.
  • ARDS is a heterogeneous process.
    ○ Includes areas of lung that contain the following
      ▪ Consolidated alveoli
      ▪ Atelectatic, but recruitable, alveoli
      ▪ Normal alveoli
  • Injured areas are usually concentrated in gravity-dependent areas of the lung, such as West zone 3 (see Chap. 3).
▶ Can also lead to systemic extra-pulmonary organ dysfunction.
  • Persistent mortality rate of 30% for patients with ARDS is usually secondary to multiple organ dysfunction as opposed to isolated respiratory failure.

Phases

▶ Exudative phase
  • First 2–7 days of the clinical course.
  • Alveolar-capillary barrier is compromised.
    ○ Loss of epithelial integrity
      ▪ Leads to intra-alveolar flooding
    ○ Injury to type II pneumocytes
      ▪ Leads to decreased fluid transport and decreased surfactant production
    ○ Loss of protective barrier
      ▪ Leads to increased risk of infection
▶ Fibroproliferative phase
  • Days 7–21 of clinical course
  • Infiltration of fibroblasts
    ○ Leads to remodeling.
    ○ Possible pathologic changes in the lung as a result of fibrosis:
      ▪ Decreased lung compliance
      ▪ Decreased functional residual capacity
      ▪ V/Q imbalances
      ▪ Increased physiologic dead space
      ▪ Severe hypoxemia

- Development of pulmonary hypertension
  - Most patients regain relatively normal function over 6–12 months after surviving the acute illness.
  - Small minority of patients retain significant long-term fibrosis.

Possible Etiologies

▶ Direct lung injury
- Common causes
  - Pneumonia
  - Aspiration
- Less common causes
  - Pulmonary contusion
  - Fat emboli
  - Near drowning
  - Inhalation injury

▶ Indirect lung injury
- Common causes
  - Sepsis
  - Severe trauma
  - Severe acute pancreatitis
- Less common causes
  - Cardiopulmonary bypass
  - Drug overdose
  - Fulminant hepatic failure
  - Transfusion reaction

Mechanisms of Ventilator-Induced Lung Injury in Acute Respiratory Distress Syndrome

▶ Volutrauma
- Refers to overdistention of alveoli
  - Leads to increased alveolar permeability, and thus can worsen intra-alveolar flooding

▶ Barotrauma
- Caused by excessively high plateau pressures (see Chap. 4)
  - Leads to increased risk of pneumothorax

▶ Cyclic opening and closing of atelectatic alveoli (see Chap. 4)
- Causes increased alveolar shearing forces and compromises epithelial integrity

SYMPTOMS AND SIGNS

Symptoms

▶ Dyspnea
▶ Fever
▶ Palpitations
▶ Mental status changes

Signs

▶ Fever
▶ Tachycardia
▶ Tachypnea
  • Shallow respirations
▶ Hypoxia
▶ Normo- or hypocarbia
▶ Crackles/rhonchi on auscultation
▶ Mental status changes

DIAGNOSIS

General

▶ History
▶ Physical examination

Definition Criteria

▶ Acute onset
▶ Bilateral diffuse alveolar infiltrates
▶ PAWP ≤ 18 mmHg
▶ Acute lung injury
  • $PaO_2:FIO_2$ ratio ≤ 300
▶ ARDS
  • $PaO_2:FIO_2$ ratio ≤ 200

Laboratory Tests

▶ ABG
  • Low, normal, or elevated pH (depends on etiology of ARDS)

- Low PaO_2
- Low or normal $PaCO_2$
▶ Radiographic tests
  - CXR
    - Bilateral diffuse alveolar infiltrates.
    - Cardiac silhouette is usually normal.
      - Helps differentiate ARDS from CHF
    - Radiographic changes often lag several hours behind changes in the clinical situation.
  - Chest computerized tomography scan
    - Bilateral diffuse alveolar infiltrates
      - Demonstrates that the injured areas are usually concentrated in dependent areas of the lung in West zone 3 (see Chap. 3)
    - Usually *not* needed to make the diagnosis

MANAGEMENT

General

▶ Treat the underlying etiology of ARDS.

Airway

▶ Ensure a stable airway.
  - Consider mechanical ventilation if necessary (see Chap. 4).

Oxygenation

▶ Optimize oxygenation (see Chap. 3).
  - Increase FIO_2.
  - Consider mechanical ventilation if necessary (see Chap. 4).

Mechanical Ventilator Strategies

High Inspired Fraction of Oxygen
▶ Avoid toxic levels (> 0.50) for prolonged periods of time.
  - Exposure of the patient to potentially toxic levels should be limited to a maximum of 12 hours.

Low Tidal Volume Ventilation
▶ Conventional ventilation techniques use Vt of approximately 10 cc/kg.
  • Leads to regional overdistention of normal alveoli because ARDS is a heterogeneous process.
    ◦ Overdistention can worsen the proinflammatory cytokine cascade.
  • Increases the plateau pressure.
    ◦ Increases the potential for barotrauma.
▶ Use Vt of approximately 4–6 cc/kg.
  • Improves survival.
  • Reduces the patient's length of time dependent on mechanical ventilation.
  • Minimizes regional overdistention of alveoli.
    ◦ Can lead to a decrease in cytokine levels.
  • Facilitates maintaining the plateau pressure < 30–35 cm H_2O (see Chap. 4).
    ◦ Minimizes potential for barotrauma.

Permitted Controlled Hypercapnia
▶ Using low Vt ventilation can reduce the MV, which can cause an increase in $PaCO_2$.
▶ Usually the benefits of low Vt ventilation outweigh the risks of elevated $PaCO_2$.
  • Using permitted controlled hypercapnia, $PaCO_2$ levels of 50–60 mmHg can usually be maintained safely while the lung recovers.
  • Contraindications to using permitted controlled hypercapnia:
    ◦ Elevated ICP (see Chap. 7)
      ▪ Elevated $PaCO_2$ can cause cerebral vasodilatation, which can lead to increased cerebral blood flow, elevated ICP, and decreased cerebral perfusion pressure (see Chap. 7).
    ◦ Severe acidemia (pH < 7.20–7.25)
      ▪ Elevated $PaCO_2$ will further decrease the pH.
      ▪ If the patient is already severely acidemic secondary to the underlying etiology of ARDS, then avoid permitted controlled hypercapnia.
        ➢ Severely acidemic patients are usually hemodynamically unstable and require vasopressor support.

        - Vasopressors generally have decreased efficacy in a severely acidemic environment.
    - Gastric bleeding
      - Relative contraindication

Positive End-Expiratory Pressure

- See Chap. 4.
- Recruits atelectatic alveoli.
  - Reduces the risk of regional overdistention.
- Minimizes cyclic opening and closing of alveoli.
  - Maintains alveoli above the lower inflection point (see Chap. 4).
  - Reduces the amount of shear stress on the alveolar wall.
- Increases FRC.
- Decreases the shunt fraction.
  - Improves V/Q matching.
  - Improves oxygenation.
- Increases mean airway pressure (Map).
  - Increased Map increases PaO_2 (see Chap. 4).
  - Improves oxygenation.
- Reduces the need for toxic levels of FIO_2.
  - Improved oxygenation with PEEP facilitates keeping the $FIO_2 < 0.50$ (50%).
- Determining the optimal amount of PEEP:
  - Keep PEEP above the lower inflection point.
    - Requires plotting an alveolar volume/pressure curve
  - Titrate to the optimal DO_2 (see Chap. 3)
    - Requires determining CO
  - In clinical practice, it is usually sufficient to increase PEEP until acceptable oxygenation is obtained at a nontoxic level of FIO_2.
    - Patients may require PEEP levels as high as 20–25 cmH_2O.
      - Theoretical concern of hemodynamic compromise with high levels of PEEP is usually not applicable here, because the severely diseased alveoli (low compliance) do not transmit the high pressure to the intra-thoracic space.
        - Can be confirmed by placing an esophageal balloon to measure intra-thoracic pressure.
        - Thus, venous return is usually not dramatically affected.

- Must be aware of increasing plateau pressures with high levels of PEEP.
  - ➢ Can potentially increase the risk of barotrauma.

Possible Strategies for Volume Control Ventilation

- ▶ Use a decelerating-wave form for air flow delivery as opposed to a square-wave form (see Chap. 4).
  - May increase the Map and thus increase the PaO_2, thereby improving oxygenation.
- ▶ Decrease the inspiratory flow rate.
  - Under normal circumstances, it is usually set at 60 L/min.
  - Decreasing the flow rate will increase the time spent for inspiration relative to expiration, although expiration still composes a greater percentage of the respiratory cycle.
    - ○ May increase the Map and thus increase the PaO_2, thereby improving oxygenation.
    - ○ May enable lowering the level of PEEP in situations in which high PEEP has caused unacceptably high plateau pressures.
    - ○ Must be cautious of the development of autoPEEP due to insufficient time for complete expiration (see Chap. 4).

Pressure Control Ventilation

- ▶ See Chap. 4.
- ▶ Usually reserved for patients that are difficult to adequately oxygenate and have dangerously high plateau pressures with the above strategies.
  - Usually accompanied with paralyzing the patient.
- ▶ May increase the Map and thus increase the PaO_2, thereby improving oxygenation.
- ▶ Plateau pressure is controlled by setting the driving pressure and level of PEEP (see Chap. 4).
- ▶ Facilitates altering the inspiration/expiration ratio because these times are directly set on the ventilator.

Inverse Ratio Ventilation

- ▶ Inspiration normally comprises a greater percentage of the respiratory cycle than expiration.
  - Normal inspiration time:expiration time ratio is 1:2.
  - For inverse ratio ventilation, the ratio is set to 1:1 or 1.5:1.0.
- ▶ Usually only used while using pressure control ventilation.

▶ Unnatural breathing pattern that usually requires sedating and paralyzing the patient.

▶ Must be cautious of inducing autoPEEP due to insufficient time for complete expiration.

Prone Positioning

▶ Proposed mechanisms of benefit:
  • Increases FRC.
  • Alters chest wall mechanics.
  • Improves V/Q matching (see Chap. 3).
    ◦ West zone 3, the area that contains the majority of diseased alveoli, becomes the new West zone 1.
    ◦ West zone 1, the area that is relatively spared of disease, becomes the new West zone 3.
    ◦ Thus, ventilation now more closely matches perfusion:
      ▪ Reduces shunt fraction
      ▪ Improves oxygenation

▶ Can improve oxygenation, although there is no proven survival benefit.
  • Can increase the $PaO_2:FIO_2$ ratio.

▶ Theoretical complications:
  • Development of pressure sores.
  • Accidental extubation.
  • Loss of venous access.
  • Displacement of chest tubes.

▶ Complications can usually be avoided with appropriate nursing care.
  • Beds are available that can provide prone positioning.

▶ The benefits of prone positioning can be obtained by keeping the patient prone for a defined period of time (e.g., 6 hours) per day.
  • Does *not* necessarily require continuous prone positioning to have a beneficial effect.

Inhaled Nitric Oxide Therapy

▶ Dilates pulmonary, but not systemic, vasculature
  • Can decrease pulmonary hypertension

▶ Increases perfusion to well-ventilated areas of the lung, thereby improving V/Q perfusion matching (see Chap. 3)
  • Can improve oxygenation and ventilation
  • No proven survival benefit in ARDS

Steroid Therapy

▶ Controversial area of management:
  • Theoretically can improve patient outcomes when given during the fibroproliferative *late* phase of ARDS (approximately 1 week into the clinical course)
    ○ May reduce inflammation and the development of fibrosis
    ○ Must monitor closely for the development of infection
▶ Possible doses:
  • 200–300 mg IV hydrocortisone QD or its equivalent for 5–7 days
  • High-dose methylprednisolone (Solu-Medrol) for approximately 1 month
    ○ Meduri protocol (to be started at the onset of the fibroproliferative phase on days 7–10 of the clinical course)
      ▪ Loading dose of 2 mg/kg
      ▪ 2 mg/kg/day from days 1 to 14
      ▪ 1 mg/kg/day from days 15 to 21
      ▪ 0.5 mg/kg/day from days 22 to 28
      ▪ 0.25 mg/kg/day on days 29 and 30
      ▪ 0.125 mg/kg/day on days 31 and 32
▶ There is no universally agreed-on steroid protocol for patients in the fibroproliferative phase of ARDS.

CHAPTER 20

CEREBRAL VASCULAR ACCIDENT (STROKE)

ABBREVIATIONS

BP: blood pressure
CHF: congestive heart failure
CPP: cerebral perfusion pressure
CSF: cerebrospinal fluid
CT: computerized tomography
DVT: deep venous thrombosis
DWI: diffusion-weighted imaging
FFP: fresh frozen plasma
ICH: intracerebral hemorrhage
ICP: intracranial pressure
INR: international normalized ratio
LP: lumbar puncture
LV: left ventricular
MAP: mean arterial pressure
MI: myocardial infarction
PE: pulmonary embolism
PFO: patent foramen ovale
PT: prothrombin time
PTT: partial thromboplastin time
SAH: subarachnoid hemorrhage

DEFINITION

Transient Ischemic Attack

▶ A sudden onset of temporary symptoms (loss of sensation, movement, speech, mental function or vision) usually lasting

minutes, sometimes hours, that occurs when the brain is deprived of oxygen-rich blood.
► Effects reverse completely after resumption of blood flow.

Cerebral Vascular Accident (Stroke)

► Loss of brain function caused by a blockage or rupture of a cerebral blood vessel that provides oxygen to the brain
  • Ischemic stroke
    ◦ Accounts for approximately 85% of all strokes
    ◦ Classification
      ▪ Thrombotic disease
        ➢ Large-vessel disease
        ➢ Small-vessel disease
      ▪ Embolic disease
      ▪ Systemic hypoperfusion
  • Hemorrhagic stroke
    ◦ Accounts for approximately 15% of all strokes
    ◦ Classification
      ▪ Intracerebral hemorrhage (ICH)
      ▪ Subarachnoid hemorrhage (SAH)

PATHOPHYSIOLOGY

Ischemic Stroke

Thrombotic Disease
► Large-vessel disease (including extracranial and intracranial vessels that supply the brain)
  • Atherosclerotic disease
    ◦ Accounts for approximately 70% of all ischemic strokes (65% of strokes from any etiology)
    ◦ Same mechanism of deposition and thrombosis as in the pathophysiology of MI (see Chap. 11)
  • Other less common causes of large-vessel disease
    ◦ Vasoconstriction (e.g., migraine)
    ◦ Arterial dissection
    ◦ Traumatic occlusion
    ◦ Fibromuscular dysplasia

► Small-vessel disease
- Occlusion of small penetrating arteries
  ○ Can be secondary to microatheroma
    ▪ Same mechanism as atherothrombosis of large vessels
  ○ Can be secondary to lipohyalinosis
    ▪ Usually secondary to chronic hypertension.
    ▪ Endothelial injury leads to the deposition of plasma proteins and eventual degeneration of the tunica media smooth muscle.
    ▪ Smooth muscle is replaced with collagenous fibers, resulting in an inelastic and narrow lumen vessel that predisposes to thrombosis.
  ○ Typically results in lacunar infarcts
    ▪ Usually involves the basal ganglia, internal capsule, thalamus, and pons

Embolic Disease
► Accounts for approximately 20% of all ischemic strokes (20% of strokes from any etiology)
► Occurs when thrombi from an extracranial location become dislodged and travel distally to occlude cerebral vessels downstream
- Thrombi as a result of atrial fibrillation account for approximately 50% of all embolic strokes.
  ○ The yearly risk of stroke from atrial fibrillation without anticoagulation is approximately 3–5%.
- Other etiologies of embolic stroke:
  ○ LV dysfunction
    ▪ Usually secondary to a previous MI or history of CHF
  ○ Valvular disease (usually the mitral valve is involved)
    ▪ Thrombus
    ▪ Calcification
    ▪ Endocarditis
  ○ Paradoxical emboli secondary to a PFO
    ▪ Venous thromboembolism crosses from the right atrium to the left atrium through a PFO.
    ▪ Patient has a stroke as opposed to a PE.
  ○ Arterial atheroemboli
    ▪ Often arise from atherosclerotic lesions in the aortic arch, carotid arteries, and vertebral arteries

Systemic Hypoperfusion
▶ Cerebral hypoperfusion and stroke can result from a combination of systemic hypotension coupled with atherosclerotic disease and/or lipohyalinosis that limits distal blood flow.
▶ This reduction in CPP causes the small arterioles to constrict in an effort to maintain pressure, thus further reducing blood flow.
▶ Watershed areas, which are areas of the brain that lie between two major vascular supplies, are most at risk for stroke during periods of systemic hypotension and decreased CPP.

Hemorrhagic Stroke

Intracerebral Hemorrhage
▶ Accounts for approximately half of all hemorrhagic strokes
▶ Most common causes
  • Hypertension
    ◦ Major cause of hemorrhage in the basal ganglia and brainstem.
    ◦ Common locations of hemorrhage include putamen/internal capsule, caudate nucleus, thalamus, pons, and cerebellum.
  • Amyloid angiopathy
    ◦ Deposition of beta amyloid sheets in the tunica media of the vessel wall causes them to become more rigid, fragile, and prone to rupture.
    ◦ Occurs mostly in elderly patients.
    ◦ Common cause of lobar hemorrhage.
▶ Other causes
  • Arteriovenous malformations
  • Neoplasms
  • Trauma
  • Use of anticoagulants (e.g., warfarin)
  • Use of thrombolytics
  • Illicit drug use (mostly amphetamines and cocaine)
  • Hemorrhagic conversion of an ischemic stroke

Subarachnoid Hemorrhage
▶ Accounts for approximately half of all hemorrhagic strokes

▶ Most common cause
  • Cerebral aneurysm rupture
    ○ Releases blood directly into the CSF under arterial pressure
▶ Less common causes
  • Arteriovenous malformations
  • Bleeding diatheses
  • Trauma
  • Amyloid angiopathy
  • Illicit drug use
▶ Potential complications
  • Vasospasm
    ○ Secondary to an interaction between the metabolites of blood and the vasculature
      ▪ Lysis of SAH blood clots releases substances that cause endothelial damage, decreased nitric oxide production (vasodilator), increased endothelin production (vasoconstrictor), and smooth muscle contraction.
    ○ Causes symptomatic ischemia and infarction in approximately 20–30% of patients with aneurysmal SAH
      ▪ Leading cause of death and disability after aneurysm rupture
    ○ Typically begins around 3 days after onset of SAH
      ▪ Peak vasospasm usually occurs approximately 7–8 days after onset of SAH.
  • Hydrocephalus
    ○ Common complication after SAH.
      ▪ Blood interferes with CSF uptake.
    ○ Spontaneous improvement occurs in approximately 50% of patients.
  • Hyponatremia
    ○ Common complication after SAH.
    ○ Likely mediated by hypothalamic injury.
      ▪ Usually secondary to syndrome of inappropriate secretion of antidiuretic hormone (SIADH) or cerebral salt wasting (see Chap. 7).
  • Cardiac abnormalities
    ○ Dysrhythmias and electrocardiographic changes
      ▪ Likely related to cardiac ischemia

- ○ Association of cardiac ischemia with SAH is multifactorial
  - ▪ Autonomic dysfunction
  - ▪ Increased myocardial oxygen demand
  - ▪ Effect of medications given during treatment of SAH
- Seizures
  - ○ Occur in approximately 3% of patients with SAH
  - ○ May lead to the development of epilepsy
    - ▪ Recurrent unprovoked seizures after hospital discharge
- Rebleeding
  - ○ Without treatment, approximately 20% of patients will rebleed within 14 days and 50% within 6 months.
  - ○ Risk of rebleeding is highest on the first day after the onset of SAH.

SYMPTOMS AND SIGNS

Symptoms

- ► Severe headache
- ► Slurred or loss of speech
- ► Loss of consciousness
- ► Cognitive deficits
- ► Limb weakness
- ► Hemiplegia
- ► Sensory loss
- ► Vertigo
- ► Diplopia or a loss of visual field
- ► Aphasia
- ► Nausea and vomiting
- ► Difficulty swallowing
- ► Classic syndromes associated with a lacunar stroke
  - Pure motor hemiparesis
  - Pure sensory syndrome
  - Ataxia hemiparesis syndrome
  - Clumsy-hand dysarthria syndrome
- ► Characteristic course of stroke subtypes
  - Ischemic (thrombotic)
    - ○ Stuttering progression with periods of improvement
  - Ischemic (embolic)
    - ○ Sudden onset with maximal neurologic deficit at the onset

- Hemorrhagic (intracerebral hemorrhage)
  - Gradual progression during minutes to hours
- Hemorrhagic (SAH)
  - Abrupt onset of a sudden, severe headache and less commonly associated with *focal* neurologic deficits

Signs

▶ Physical examination reveals one, or some combination, of the above neurologic symptoms.

▶ Fever.

▶ Hypertension.

▶ Hypotension.

▶ Atrial fibrillation.

▶ Murmur on auscultation.

▶ Evidence of peripheral artery disease.
  - Carotid artery bruits
  - Lower extremity hypoperfusion

DIAGNOSIS

General

▶ History

▶ Physical examination

Conditions That Can Mimic Stroke

▶ Hyperglycemia

▶ Hypoglycemia

▶ Seizure

▶ Multiple sclerosis

▶ Hyperventilation

▶ Tumor

▶ Complicated migraine

Laboratory Tests

▶ No specific tests are needed to make the diagnosis of stroke, but they can help identify possible precipitating factors:
  - Complete blood count, including platelets.
  - Electrolytes (basic metabolic panel).

- Serum glucose.
- Liver function tests.
- PT, INR, and PTT.
- Toxicology screen.
- Consider an evaluation for hypercoagulable states (see Chap. 18) in patients without any apparent stroke risk factors.

Electrocardiogram

▶ Assess for evidence of a previous MI.
▶ Assess for the presence of atrial fibrillation.

Radiographic Tests

Assessing for Presence of Stroke
▶ CT scan (without IV contrast):
  - Rapid study that can be obtained in a timely manner.
  - Highly sensitive for the diagnosis of hemorrhagic stroke.
    ○ Mostly used in the immediate acute setting to exclude hemorrhage.
  - May not be able to detect small strokes.
  - May not be able to differentiate acute from previous strokes.
  - Radiographic changes may lag behind the clinical picture.
    ○ Sensitivity for diagnosing ischemic stroke increases after 24 hours of the onset of symptoms.
▶ Magnetic resonance imaging:
  - Time needed to perform the examination is longer than CT.
    ○ More limited by patient contraindications and intolerance compared to CT.
  - More sensitive than CT for the *early* diagnosis of brain infarction.
    ○ DWI and fluid-attenuated inversion recovery images can often identify small strokes that are missed on CT.
  - DWI can usually differentiate acute from previous strokes.

Assessing the Cerebral Vasculature
▶ CT angiography
  - Noninvasive
  - Rapid acquisition of images

- Exposes the patient to IV contrast dye and its potential nephrotoxicity
▶ Magnetic resonance angiography
  - Noninvasive
  - May overestimate the presence and degree of stenosis
  - Exposes the patient to IV contrast dye (gadolinium)
    ○ Less toxic profile compared to CT contrast dye
▶ Transcranial Doppler
  - Noninvasive
  - Can be performed at the bedside
  - Operator dependent
  - Can detect the presence of vasospasm
  - Less sensitive for the vertebrobasilar (posterior) circulation
▶ Cerebral angiography
  - Invasive
  - Exposes the patient to IV contrast dye and its potential nephrotoxicity
  - Gold standard test for imaging the circulation
    ○ Rarely used in the diagnosis of acute stroke
      ▪ More commonly used for the diagnosis of vasospasm
    ○ Often needed for instituting various treatments

Assessing for the Etiology of Embolic Ischemic Stroke
▶ Duplex ultrasonography of bilateral carotid arteries
  - Noninvasive
  - Assesses for the presence and degree of carotid stenosis
▶ Magnetic resonance angiography of the carotid arteries
  - Assesses for the presence and degree of carotid stenosis
  - Can also visualize the vertebral arteries, which are difficult to assess with duplex ultrasonography
▶ Transthoracic echocardiography
  - Noninvasive
  - Assesses for the presence of a cardioembolic source
  - Can be a limited study for the assessment of the cardiac valves, left atrial appendage, aortic arch, and PFO
▶ Transesophageal echocardiography
  - Invasive
    ○ Requires administering sedatives to the patient
  - Assesses for the presence of a cardioembolic source

- Superior to transthoracic echocardiography in assessing the cardiac valves, left atrial appendage, aortic arch, and a PFO
▶ Lower extremity duplex ultrasonography
  - If a PFO is detected on echocardiography, consider assessing for a lower extremity DVT.

Lumbar Puncture (LP)

▶ Consider LP when there is a strong suspicion of SAH despite normal radiographic imaging (CT or magnetic resonance imaging).
▶ Must ensure there is no evidence of elevated ICP that can predispose the patient to brainstem herniation on LP.
▶ Presence of xanthochromia (pink or yellow tint) represents hemoglobin degradation products and indicates that blood has been in the CSF for at least 2 hours.
  - May help differentiate between SAH and a traumatic LP.

MANAGEMENT

Airway

▶ Ensure a secure airway.
  - Consider mechanical ventilation if necessary (see Chap. 4).
    - Glasgow Coma Scale score ≤ 8 is an indication for intubation.

Ischemic Stroke

Etiology
▶ Attempt to determine the etiology.
  - Thrombotic
    - Large-vessel vs. small-vessel disease
  - Embolic
    - Source of embolus
  - Systemic hypoperfusion

Thrombolytic Therapy
▶ Indications:
  - Clinical diagnosis is ischemic stroke.
    - No evidence of a hemorrhagic component.

- Onset of symptoms within 3 hours of the initiation of treatment.
  - If the exact time of onset is unknown, it is defined as the last time the patient was witnessed to be normal.
▶ Contraindications:
  - Historical
    - Stroke or head trauma within the past 3 months
    - History of ICH
    - Major surgery within the past 14 days
    - Gastrointestinal or genitourinary bleeding within the previous 3 weeks
    - MI within the past 3 months
    - Arterial puncture at a noncompressible site within the past 7 days
    - LP within the past 7 days
  - Clinical
    - Rapidly improving stroke symptoms
    - Only minor neurologic signs
    - Seizure with postictal residual neurologic deficits
    - Symptoms suggestive of SAH, even if radiographic tests are normal
    - Concurrent acute MI
    - Persistent hypertension with systolic BP > 185 mmHg, diastolic BP > 110 mmHg, or requiring aggressive therapy to control the BP
    - Pregnancy or lactation
    - Active bleeding or acute trauma
  - Laboratory
    - Platelets < 100,000/mm^3
    - Serum glucose < 50 mg/dl or > 400 mg/dl
    - INR > 1.5
    - Elevated PTT to > 1.5 times normal
  - Radiographic
    - Evidence of hemorrhage
    - Evidence of major infarct signs, including diffuse swelling, parenchymal hypodensity, and/or effacement of > 33% of the middle cerebral artery territory
▶ ICH is the most severe complication.
  - Infusion should be stopped immediately.
  - Consider administering platelets, FFP, or cryoprecipitate to help stop the bleeding (see Chap. 6).

▶ Alteplase (Activase, t-PA):
  • Only thrombolytic medication that is approved by the U.S. Food and Drug Administration for the treatment of ischemic stroke.
    ◦ Patients were shown to be 30% more likely to experience an excellent recovery at 3 months compared to patients treated with placebo.
    ◦ Still has undesirably high rates of reocclusion (34%) and neurologic deterioration after initial clinical improvement.
  • Dose:
    ◦ 0.9 mg/kg IV (maximum, 90 mg) infused over 60 minutes.
      ▪ 10% of the total dose should be administered as an IV bolus over the first minute.
    ◦ Intra-arterial route can also be used.
      ▪ Thrombolysis is performed under direct angiographic visualization.
      ▪ Requires approximately one-third of the IV dose.
    ◦ Other antithrombotic medications (heparin, warfarin, antiplatelet agents) should not be administered, and invasive procedures should be avoided, for at least 24 hours after the alteplase infusion is completed.
    ◦ Patients should undergo a follow-up non-contrast head CT scan before reinstituting other anti-thrombotic medications.

Antiplatelet Medications
▶ Aspirin
  • Only antiplatelet medication that has been evaluated for the treatment of ischemic stroke
    ◦ Shown to reduce the risk of early recurrent stroke and improve long-term outcome without a major risk of hemorrhagic complications
  • Dose
    ◦ 160–325 mg PO/NG QD.
    ◦ Start therapy within 48 hours of the onset of symptoms.
      ▪ Exceptions include patients who are receiving alteplase thrombolytic therapy, IV heparin, or oral anticoagulants (e.g., warfarin).
▶ Glycoprotein Ia antagonists
  • May be used as alternatives for patients who are intolerant to aspirin

- Dose
  - Clopidogrel (Plavix): 75 mg PO/NG QD
  - Ticlopidine (Ticlid): 250 mg PO/NG BID
  - Dipyridamole (Persantine): 75–100 mg PO/NG QID
▶ Glycoprotein IIb/IIIa antagonists
  - Currently under evaluation for the treatment of acute ischemic stroke

Heparin and Low-Molecular-Weight Heparin
▶ Early anticoagulation with heparin and low-molecular-weight heparin has not been shown to provide a benefit in unselected patients with acute ischemic stroke.
  - Limited efficacy.
  - Increased risk of bleeding complications.
▶ May consider administering early anticoagulation in selected patients with cardioembolic and large-artery ischemic strokes and for progressing thromboembolic strokes.
  - Aspirin should still be considered the antithrombotic agent of first choice.
▶ Dose:
  - Heparin:
    - 10–12 U/kg IV q hour as a continuous infusion.
    - Do *not* administer a bolus dose.
    - Titrate dose to a PTT of 1.5–2.5 times normal value.
  - Enoxaparin (Lovenox): 1 mg/kg SC q 12 hours.

Hemorrhagic Stroke

Anti-Thrombotic Medications
▶ All anti-thrombotic medications (thrombolytics, antiplatelet agents, heparin, low-molecular-weight heparin, warfarin) are *contraindicated*.
  - Correct any coagulopathies.

Specific Considerations for Managing Subarachnoid Hemorrhage
▶ Treatment of aneurysms
  - Surgical therapy
    - Involves placing a clip across the neck of the aneurysm

- Endovascular therapy
  - Involves placing coils into the lumen of the aneurysm, thereby inducing thrombosis and obliterating the aneurysmal sac
- Timing of intervention
  - Remains an area of controversy
  - Advantages of early intervention (within 48–72 hours of SAH)
    - Reduces the risk of rebleeding
    - Facilitates the aggressive management of vasospasm (see below)
  - Disadvantages of early intervention
    - More technically challenging due to the presence of edema
    - May be associated with an increased risk of ischemic complications
  - Delayed intervention is usually instituted around 10–14 days after SAH
▶ Vasospasm
- Calcium channel blockers
  - Nimodipine (Nimotop)
    - 60 mg PO/NG q 4 hours
    - Initiate therapy within 3–4 days of the SAH
    - May help prevent the onset of vasospasm
- Magnesium sulfate ($MgSO_4$)
  - This treatment modality is based on efficacy in treating preeclampsia/eclampsia
  - May help prevent the onset of vasospasm
- "Triple-H" therapy
  - Components
    - Hemodilution
    - Hypertension (can use pressor agents such as phenylephrine or dopamine) (see Chap. 6)
    - Hypervolemia (can use crystalloid or colloid solutions – avoid using hetastarch and dextran due to potential antiplatelet effects) (see Chap. 6)
  - Should only be instituted after the aneurysm has been treated with either surgical or endovascular therapy
  - Intended to increase MAP, and thereby increase CPP

- Other treatment modalities to consider for refractory vasospasm (preferable to institute these therapies after the aneurysm has already been treated)
  - Intra-arterial papaverine therapy
    - Administered at the time of angiogram
  - Percutaneous intra-arterial angioplasty
    - Performed at the time of angiogram
  - Intrathecal nitroprusside (Nipride)
▶ Hydrocephalus
- Consider placing a ventriculostomy drain (see Chap. 7)
  - Provides the added benefit of being able to measure ICP

General Management Principles

Blood Pressure
▶ Ischemic stroke
- Elevated BP is usually a natural compensation that is necessary to maintain an adequate CPP in the setting of an obstructed vessel.
  - Lowering the BP has been associated with neurologic deterioration.
- Recommendations:
  - Elevated BP should not be treated unless the hypertension is extreme (systolic BP > 200 mmHg, diastolic BP > 110 mmHg).
    - Labetalol is the first-choice anti-hypertensive (see Chap. 6).
    - Nitroprusside/nitroglycerin are second-choice anti-hypertensives (see Chap. 6).
  - Maintain systolic BP ≥ 130–140 mmHg.
    - May use phenylephrine or norepinephrine if necessary (see Chap. 6).
▶ Hemorrhagic stroke
- Elevated BP can increase the risk for rebleeding.
- Lowering the BP can increase the risk of infarction.
  - ICH can elevate the ICP.
  - Lowering the BP can lower the CPP, thereby increasing the risk of ischemia and infarction.

- Recommendations:
  - Maintain the systolic BP between approximately 140 and 170 mmHg.
    - Use labetalol, nitroprusside, nitroglycerin, phenylephrine, and norepinephrine as necessary (see Chap. 6).
  - Monitor the patient closely for signs of cerebral hypoperfusion.
  - Consider placing an invasive ICP monitor to facilitate titrating the BP to maintain the CPP at approximately 65–70 mmHg (see Chap. 7).

Maintain Normoglycemia
▶ See Chap. 7.
▶ Hyperglycemia (> 108 mg/dl) can augment brain injury and worsen functional outcomes.
- May increase tissue acidosis from anaerobic metabolism.
- May increase free radical production.
- May further compromise the blood–brain barrier.

Maintain Normothermia
▶ See Chap. 7.
▶ Hyperthermia can augment brain injury and worsen functional outcomes.
- May increase the release of neurotransmitters.
- May increase oxygen radical production.
- May further compromise the blood–brain barrier.

Correct Metabolic Derangements
▶ Electrolyte abnormalities
▶ SIADH, diabetes insipidus, or cerebral salt wasting (see Chap. 7)

Consider Obtaining a Swallowing Function Evaluation before Reinstituting Oral Feeding
▶ Strict aspiration precautions should be maintained.

Administer Stress Ulcer Prophylaxis
▶ See Chap. 10.

▶ Consider continuing antisecretory therapy even when the patient is being fed secondary to increased acid secretion.

Administer Deep Venous Thrombosis Prophylaxis
▶ See Chap. 10.
▶ Pulmonary embolism is the most common cause of death during the 2–4 weeks after an acute stroke.
▶ For patients with hemorrhagic strokes and/or contraindications to antithrombotic therapy:
   • Apply intermittent pneumatic compression devices.
   • Consider placing a temporary inferior vena cava filter.

SUGGESTED READINGS

Hall JB, Schmidt GA, Wood LDH. *Principles of Critical Care*. 2nd ed. New
    York: McGraw-Hill, 1998.
Marino PL. *The ICU Book*. 2nd ed. Philadelphia: Williams & Wilkins, 1998.
The Cleveland Clinic medical education disease management online pro-
gram. http://www.clevelandclinicmeded.com/diseasemanagement.

INDEX

NOTE: Page numbers followed by *f* indicate figures; those followed by *t* indicate tables.

A

Abciximab in myocardial infarction, 119
Acetaminophen, liver failure from, 176, 182
Acetazolamide in metabolic alkalosis, 89
N-Acetylcysteine in acetaminophen toxicity, 183
Acid–base disorders, 79–91
Acidemia, 80
Acidosis
  anion gap
    increased, mnemonic for, 85t
    normal, 83–84
  hyperchloremic, 83–84
  metabolic, 80t, 83–87
    compensation in, 81t
    in sepsis, 151
  osmolar gap, 85–87
  renal tubular, 83–84
  respiratory, 80t, 89–90
    acute, 81t
    chronic, 81t
  treatment, 90
ACTH in sepsis, 155
Activase. *See* Alteplase
Acute respiratory distress syndrome (ARDS), 197–206
  cytokines in, 198
  definition, 197, 200
  diagnosis, 200–201
  exudative phase, 198
  fibroproliferative phase, 198–199
  inhaled nitric oxide in, 205
  in liver failure, 174, 180
  management, 201–206
  mechanical ventilation in, 201–205
    inspired fraction of oxygen in, 201
    inverse ratio in, 204–205
    low tidal volume in, 202
    permitted controlled hypercapnia in, 202–203
    positive end-expiratory pressure in, 203–204
    pressure control in, 204
    volume control in, 204
  pathophysiology, 198–199
  possible etiologies, 199
  prone positioning in, 205
  in sepsis, 154
  in severe acute pancreatitis, 168
  steroid therapy in, 206
  symptoms and signs, 200
  ventilator-induced lung injury in, 199
Acyclovir in herpes simplex virus infection, 184
Adrenal insufficiency, shock in, 12
α_1-Adrenergic receptor, 54
α_2-Adrenergic receptor, 54
  agonists
    clonidine, 59
    dexmedetomidine hydrochloride, 61
β_1-Adrenergic receptor, 54
  blockers, 59. *See also* Beta-blockers
β_2-Adrenergic receptor, 54
  agonists in COPD, 136
Adrenocorticotropic hormone in sepsis, 155
Aggrastat in myocardial infarction, 119
Airway management
  in acute respiratory distress syndrome, 201
  in heart failure, 128
  in myocardial infarction, 118
  in pneumonia, 143
  in sepsis, 151
  in severe acute pancreatitis, 166
  in strokes, 216
  in venous thromboembolism, 192

Albuterol in COPD, 136
  ipratropium with, 136
Alcohol ingestion
  osmolar gap from isopropyl alcohol, 85
  severe acute pancreatitis from, 159–160
Aldactone in heart failure, 130
Aldosterone antagonists in heart failure, 130
Alkalemia, 80
Alkalosis
  metabolic, 80t, 87–89
    compensation in, 81t
  respiratory, 80t, 90–91
    acute, 81t
    chronic, 81t
    treatment, 91
Alteplase
  in ischemic stroke, 218
  in myocardial infarction, 121
  in venous thromboembolism, 196
Alveolar-arterial diffusion gradient, 19
Alveoli
  collapse, 33
  compliance curve, 35, 36f
  pressure in lung zones, 49t
AmBisome in sepsis, 153
γ-Aminobutyric acid (GABA) receptor, 55
Aminoglycosides in pneumonia, 145
Aminophylline, intravenous, in COPD, 136
5-Aminosalicylic acid, severe acute pancreatitis from, 160
Ammonia levels in hepatic encephalopathy, 172–173
Amoxicillin in COPD, 136
Amphotericin B in sepsis, 153
  liposomal form in, 153
Ampicillin/sulbactam in pneumonia, 145
Amylase levels in severe acute pancreatitis
  serum levels, 163–164
  urine levels, 164
Amyloid angiopathy, intracerebral hemorrhage in, 210
Analgesics and sedatives, 60–62
Anaphylactic shock, 12
Aneurysm
  cerebral, ruptured, subarachnoid hemorrhage in, 211
  management in hemorrhagic strokes, 219–220
Angiography
  pulmonary, in pulmonary embolism, 192
  in strokes, 214–215

Angiopathy, amyloid, intracerebral hemorrhage in, 210
Angioplasty, percutaneous intra-arterial, in vasospasm, 221
Angiotensin-converting enzyme inhibitors
  in heart failure, 129
  in myocardial infarction, 120
Angiotensin II receptor blockers in heart failure, 130
Anion gap
  acidosis
    increased, mnemonic for, 85t
    normal, 83–84
  decreased, 82
  equation for, 79, 81
  increased, 82
  normal, 82
Antibiotics
  in COPD, 136
  in liver failure, 181
  in sepsis, 151–152
  in severe acute pancreatitis, 168
  severe acute pancreatitis from, 160
Anticholinergic therapy in COPD, 136
Antidiuretic hormone secretion, inappropriate
  in cerebral vascular accident, 222
  in head injuries, 69
Antihypertensives, 58–59
Antiinflammatory agents, severe acute pancreatitis from, 160
Antiplatelet medications in ischemic stroke, 218
Antithrombin in sepsis, 149
α₁-Antitrypsin deficiency in emphysema, 134
Aorta
  balloon pump in myocardial infarction, 123
  pressure rule of fives, 46t
ARDS. See Acute respiratory distress syndrome (ARDS)
5-ASA, severe acute pancreatitis from, 160
L-Asparaginase, severe acute pancreatitis from, 160
Aspiration, pulmonary, in enteral nutrition, 98–99
Aspirin
  in ischemic stroke, 218
  in myocardial infarction, 118
Assist control ventilation, 38–39, 39t
Atelectasis, 33
Atherosclerosis
  ischemic strokes in, 208
  myocardial infarction in, 116

Ativan, 61
Atmospheric pressure, 18
Atrial pressure. *See* Right atrial pressure
AutoPEEP, 37–38
  and mechanical ventilation, 38
  and pulmonary capillary wedge
    pressure, 51
Avapro in heart failure, 130
Azactam in pneumonia, 145
Azathioprine, severe acute pancreatitis
    from, 160
Azithromycin in pneumonia, 145
Aztreonam in pneumonia, 145

B
Balloon pump, intra-aortic, in myocar-
    dial infarction, 123
Barbiturate coma in head injuries,
    76–77
Base
  deficit, 81
  excess, 81
Bedside placement of feeding tubes,
    95–96
Benzodiazepines, 60–61
  toxicity reversal with flumazenil, 60
Beta-blockers, 59
  in heart failure, 130
  in myocardial infarction, 120
Biaxin in pneumonia, 145
Bicarbonate levels
  in acidosis, 80t
  in alkalosis, 80t
  deficiency of, hyperchloremic acido-
    sis from, 83–84
  excess of, metabolic alkalosis from,
    87–88
  ideal value, 18, 24
  normal range, 80
Bicarbonate therapy
  in anion gap acidemia, 86
  contraindications, 83
  in renal tubular acidosis, 84
Bi-level positive airway pressure, 40, 40t
Blood
  cultures in pneumonia, 143
  gases, arterial. *See also* Carbon dioxi-
    ide; Oxygen
    in acute respiratory distress syn-
      drome, 200–201
    in pulmonary embolism, 190–191
  products, 62–65
    cryoprecipitate, 64
    fresh frozen plasma, 64
    in liver failure, 181–182
    packed red blood cells, 62–63
    platelets, 63

  tests
    in myocardial infarction, 118, 118t
    in pneumonia, 142
Blood pressure
  factors affecting, 3–6
  in hemorrhagic stroke, 221–222
  hypertension
    intracerebral hemorrhage in, 210
    medications in, 58–59
  in ischemic stroke, 221
  in sepsis, 151
Blue bloater, 133
Bohr effect, 20–21, 20f
Brevibloc, 59
Bronchitis, chronic, 133, 134
Bronchodilators in COPD, 136
Bronchoscopic testing in pneumonia, 143
Budd-Chiari syndrome, 177, 183
Bumetanide in heart failure, 131
Bumex in heart failure, 131

C
Calcium
  channel blockers in hemorrhagic
    strokes, 220
  hypercalcemia causing severe acute
    pancreatitis, 160
  in parenteral nutrition, 101t
  severe acute pancreatitis from, 161
Calorimetry, indirect, 105
Capacity of lungs, subdivisions of, 30f
Capoten. *See* Captopril
Captopril
  in heart failure, 129
  in myocardial infarction, 120
Carafate in stress ulcer prophylaxis, 110
Carbapenems in pneumonia, 145
Carbohydrates in parenteral nutrition,
    100
Carbon dioxide
  alveolar partial pressure, 25
  arterial partial pressure, 18, 24, 25
    in acidosis, 80t
    in acute respiratory distress syn-
      drome, 201
    in alkalosis, 80t
    in head injuries, 75
    normal, 80
    in pulmonary embolism, 190
  fraction of alveolar gas, 25
Carbon monoxide diffusing capacity in
    COPD, 135
Cardiac cycle
  diastolic and systolic pressures in, 9f,
    9–10
  differential diagnosis of dysfunction
    in, 10

Cardiac failure. *See* Heart failure, congestive
Cardiac index
  equation for, 46
  pulmonary artery catheter measurements, 51t
Cardiac ischemia in subarachnoid hemorrhage, 211–212
Cardiac output
  cardiac cycle in, 9f, 9–10
  central factors in, 4–5
  contractility affecting, 5, 6, 7f
  heart rate affecting, 4, 5f
  humoral factors in, 5–6
  measurement with Fick equation, 49
  peripheral factors in, 5
  pressure and volume relationships in, 6–10, 7f
  in shock, 12, 13, 13t
  Starling curve in, 8f, 8–9
  thermodilution measurements, 48–49
    potential errors in, 49t, 49
Cardiogenic shock, 11, 13
Cardiovascular system
  in liver failure, 173, 180
  response in shock, 12
  in sepsis, 149, 151
Carvedilol in heart failure, 130
Catapres, 59
Catheters
  pulmonary artery, 45–52. *See also* Pulmonary artery catheters (Swan-Ganz)
  thrombus from, cardiac output measurement in, 49t
Cefotan in pneumonia, 145
Cefotetan in pneumonia, 145
Cefoxitin in pneumonia, 145
Ceftazidime in pneumonia, 145
Ceftin in pneumonia, 145
Ceftriaxone in pneumonia, 145
Cefuroxime in pneumonia, 145
Central nervous system
  in hepatic encephalopathy, 172–173, 179
  response in shock, 12
Central venous pressure
  normal pressure, 46t
  rule of fives, 46t
  in venous thromboembolism, 195
  waveform, 47f
Cephalosporins in pneumonia, 145
Cerebral blood flow, and mean arterial pressure, 71, 72f
Cerebral edema in hepatic encephalopathy, 173, 179

Cerebral perfusion pressure
  in embolic strokes, 210
  equation for, 68
  and mean arterial pressure in head injury, 71–72, 72f
Cerebral vascular accident, 207–223
  blood pressure control in, 221–222
  conditions mimicking stroke, 213
  definition, 208
  diagnosis, 213–216
  electrocardiography in, 213–214
  general management principles in, 221–223
  hemorrhagic stroke, 208, 210–212
    management, 219–221
    symptoms, 213
  ischemic stroke, 208–210
    management, 216–219
    symptoms, 212–213
  laboratory tests, 213–214
  management, 216–223
  pathophysiology, 208–212
  radiographic tests, 214–216
    for cerebral vasculature assessment, 214–215
    for etiology of embolic ischemic stroke, 215–216
    for presence of stroke, 214
  symptoms and signs, 212–213
  transient ischemic attack in, 207–208
Cerebrospinal fluid in head injuries, 74
Chest films
  in acute respiratory distress syndrome, 201
  in COPD, 135
  in heart failure, 128
  in pneumonia, 142
  in pulmonary embolism, 191
  in severe acute pancreatitis, 165
Chest physiotherapy in COPD, 136
Chills
  in pneumonia, 142
  in sepsis, 149
Chloride in parenteral nutrition, 101t
Cholangiopancreatography
  endoscopic retrograde
    in gallstone pancreatitis, 169–170
    severe acute pancreatitis from, 162
  magnetic resonance, in severe acute pancreatitis, 165
Cholecystitis, acalculous, in parenteral nutrition, 104
Chronic obstructive pulmonary disease. *See* COPD (chronic obstructive pulmonary disease)
Cipro in pneumonia, 145
Ciprofloxacin in pneumonia, 145

Cisatracurium, 62
   in head injuries, 76
Clarithromycin in pneumonia, 145
Cleocin in pneumonia, 145
Clindamycin in pneumonia, 145
Clonidine, 59
Clopidogrel
   in ischemic stroke, 219
   in myocardial infarction, 119
Closing volume, and functional residual capacity, 32f, 32–33
Coagulation
   disseminated intravascular, in head injuries, 70
   hypercoagulable states, 186
   in liver failure, 175, 181–182
   in sepsis, 148
Collecting duct, 82–83
Coma induction in head injuries, 76–77
Combivent in COPD, 136
Community-acquired pneumonia, 139–145
Compensation, metabolic or respiratory, 81t
Computerized tomography
   in acute respiratory distress syndrome, 201
   in intracranial pressure increase, 68
   in liver failure, 178
   in severe acute pancreatitis, 165–166
   spiral, in pulmonary embolism, 192
   in strokes, 214
Continuous positive airway pressure (CPAP), in weaning from ventilator, 43–44
Contractility, and cardiac output, 5, 6, 7f
COPD (chronic obstructive pulmonary disease), 133–137
   antibiotics in, 136
   bronchodilators in, 136
   chest physiotherapy in, 136
   corticosteroids in, 137
   definition, 133
   diagnosis, 134–135
   management, 135–137
   noninvasive positive pressure or mechanical ventilation in, 136, 137
   oxygen therapy in, 135–136
   pathophysiology, 133–134
   symptoms and signs, 134
Coreg in heart failure, 130
Coronary arteries in myocardial infarction, 116
Corticosteroids. *See* Steroid therapy

Cough
   in COPD, 134–135
   in pneumonia, 142
Coumadin in deep venous thrombosis prophylaxis, 109
Cozaar in heart failure, 130
Creatinine phosphokinase levels in myocardial infarction, 118t
Cryoprecipitate, 64
Crystalloid intravenous fluids, 65t, 65–66
Cullen sign in severe acute pancreatitis, 163
Cushing triad in intracranial pressure increase, 68
Cystic fibrosis, severe acute pancreatitis in, 162
Cytokines, proinflammatory
   in sepsis, 148–149
   in severe acute pancreatitis, 158

D
D-dimer test in deep venous thrombosis, 189
Dalteparin
   in deep venous thrombosis prophylaxis, 109
   in myocardial infarction, 121
Dead space, 25
   anatomic, 25
   calculation of, 24
   hypercarbia in, 26
   physiologic, 25
   in pulmonary embolism, 187
   total, 25
Deep venous thrombosis, 185, 186
   prophylaxis in cerebral vascular accident, 223
Demadex in heart failure, 131
Depakote, severe acute pancreatitis from, 160
Dexamethasone dosage compared to other steroids, 15t
Dexmedetomidine hydrochloride, 61
Dextran, 66
Diabetes insipidus
   central, in head injuries, 69–70
   in cerebral vascular accident, 222
Dialysis in anion gap acidosis, 86
Diaphoresis in sepsis, 150
Diastolic volume or pressure. *See* End diastolic volume
Didanosine, severe acute pancreatitis from, 160
Diflucan in sepsis, 152
Digoxin in heart failure, 130
Dilaudid, 60
Diovan in heart failure, 130

Dipyridamole
  in ischemic stroke, 219
  in myocardial infarction, 119
Disseminated intravascular coagulation
      in head injuries, 70
Diuretics
  in heart failure, 130–131
  severe acute pancreatitis from, 160
Dobbhoff tube, 94–95
Dobutamine, 56t, 57
  in heart failure, 131
  in liver failure, 180
  in myocardial infarction, 122
  in sepsis, 154
  in severe acute pancreatitis, 168
  in venous thromboembolism, 195
Dopamine, 56t, 57
  in liver failure, 180
  in myocardial infarction, 122
  in sepsis, 154
  in severe acute pancreatitis, 167
  in venous thromboembolism, 195
D_1-Dopamine receptor, 54–55
D_2-Dopamine receptor, 55
Doppler ultrasonography, transcranial,
      in strokes, 215
Doxycycline in COPD, 136
Drotrecogin alfa in sepsis, 155
Drug-induced conditions
  hyperchloremic acidosis, 84
  liver failure, 176
  severe acute pancreatitis, 160–161
Duodenal feeding, 94–95
Dyspnea
  in acute respiratory distress syn-
      drome, 200
  in COPD, 134–135
  in pneumonia, 142

E
Echocardiography
  in heart failure, 128
  in myocardial infarction, 118
  in pulmonary embolism, 192
  in strokes, 215–216
Edecrin in heart failure, 131
Edema, cerebral, in hepatic encepha-
      lopathy, 173, 179
Electrocardiogram
  in cerebral vascular accident, 214
  in heart failure, 128
  in myocardial infarction, 117
  in pulmonary embolism, 190
Electrolytes
  abnormalities in parenteral nutri-
      tion, 104
  dosage in parenteral nutrition, 101

Embolic strokes, 209–210
Embolism, pulmonary, 186, 187. *See
      also* Pulmonary embolism
Emphysema, 133–134
Enalapril in heart failure, 129
Encephalopathy, hepatic, 172–173
  management of, 179
End diastolic volume
  left ventricular relation to LV end
      diastolic pressure, 7f, 7–8
  relation to stroke volume, 8f, 8–9
End expiration, pulmonary capillary
      wedge pressure in, 50, 50f
End-expiratory pressure, positive,
      35–37. *See also* Positive end-
      expiratory pressure (PEEP)
Endoscopic placement of feeding tubes,
      96
Enoxaparin
  in deep venous thrombosis prophy-
      laxis, 109
  in ischemic stroke, 219
  in myocardial infarction, 121
Enteral nutrition, 93–99
  advantages, 93
  contraindications, 94
  duodenal, 94–95
  feeding tubes used in, 94–95
  formulas in
    osmolarity of, 97
    types of, 98
    volume of, 97
  gastric, 94
  jejunal, 95
  placement of feeding tubes in, 95–97
    bedside, 95–96
    endoscopic, 96
    radiographic, 96
    surgical, 97
  risk of pulmonary aspiration in,
      98–99
Epinephrine, 56, 56t
Eplerenone in heart failure, 130
Eptifibatide in myocardial infarction,
      119
Esmolol, 59
Estrogen supplements, severe acute
      pancreatitis from, 161
Ethacrynic acid in heart failure, 131
Ethylene glycol ingestion, osmolar gap
      from, 85
Expiratory reserve volume, 30t

F
Factor V Leiden, and deep venous
      thrombosis, 107, 186
Factor VIIIa transfusions, 64

Fats in parenteral nutrition, 100–101
Fatty liver of pregnancy, acute, 184
Feeding tubes, 94–95
Fentanyl, 60
Fever
  in acute respiratory distress syndrome, 200
  in cerebral vascular accident, 222
  in head injuries, 74
  in pneumonia, 142
  in sepsis, 149, 150
Fick equation, 18, 22
  for cardiac output measurement, 49
Flagyl in pneumonia, 145
"Floating swan" waveform, 48f
Florinef in sepsis, 155
Fluconazole in sepsis, 152
Fludrocortisone in sepsis, 155
Fluid resuscitation
  in liver failure, 180
  in sepsis, 153
  in severe acute pancreatitis, 167
  in venous thromboembolism, 195
Fluids
  crystalloid intravenous, 65t, 65–66
  restriction in head injuries, 73–74
Flumazenil for benzodiazepine toxicity reversal, 61
Fluoroquinolones in pneumonia, 145
Fomepizole in anion gap acidosis, 86
Formulas used in enteral nutrition, 97–98
Fortaz in pneumonia, 145
Fragmin. See Dalteparin
Functional residual capacity
  and closing volume, 32f, 32–33
  prone positioning affecting, 205
Fungemia in sepsis, treatment of, 152
Fungizone in sepsis, 152
Fungus infections, liver failure in, 181
Furosemide
  in heart failure, 131
  severe acute pancreatitis from, 160

G
Gallstone pancreatitis, 159
  management of, 169–170
Garamycin in pneumonia, 145
Gastric feeding, 94
  in stress ulcer prophylaxis, 110
Gastrointestinal tract
  in liver failure, 174, 181
  response in shock, 12
Gastrojejunostomy tube, 95
Gastrostomy tube, 94
Genitourinary system response in shock, 12

Gentamicin in pneumonia, 145
Gentran, 66
Glasgow Coma Scale, 68
  in strokes, 216
Glucose levels
  in cerebral vascular accident, 222
  in head injuries, 74
  hyperglycemia in parenteral nutrition, 103–104
  in sepsis, 154
  in severe acute pancreatitis, 168
Glycoprotein antagonists
  in ischemic stroke, 218–219
  in myocardial infarction, 119
Grey-Turner sign in severe acute pancreatitis, 163

H
Haldol, 61–62
Haloperidol, 61–62
Hampton hump in pulmonary embolism, 191
Harris Benedict formula, 105
HCTZ in heart failure, 131
Head injuries, 67–77
  central diabetes insipidus in, 69–70
  cerebral salt wasting in, 70
  cerebrospinal fluid in, 74
  clinical correlation, 77
  disseminated intravascular coagulation in, 70
  fluid restriction in, 73–74
  glucose levels in, 74
  head positioning in, 72–73
  hyperventilation in, 75
  inappropriate antidiuretic hormone secretion in, 69
  intracranial pressure increase in, 68–69
  maintenance of cerebral perfusion pressure in, 71–72
  mannitol in, 73
  paralytic agents in, 76
  pentobarbital coma in, 76–77
  sedation in, 76
  temperature regulation in, 74
  treatment of, 71–77
Heart failure, congestive, 125–132
  aldosterone antagonists in, 130
  angiotensin-converting enzyme inhibitors in, 129
  angiotensin II receptor blockers in, 130
  beta-blockers in, 130
  definition, 125–126
  diagnosis, 128
  digoxin in, 130

diuretics in, 130–131
  intravenous inotropes and vasodila-
    tors in, 131
  invasive therapies in, 132
  management, 128–132
  pathophysiology, 126–127
  symptoms and signs, 127–128
HELLP syndrome, 184
Hematologic disorders
  in liver failure, 175, 181–182
  in sepsis, 151
Hemorrhage
  intracerebral, 210
    from thrombolytic therapy,
      217–218
  subarachnoid, 210–212
    management of, 219–221
Hemorrhagic stroke, 208, 210–212
  blood pressure control in, 221–222
  intracerebral hemorrhage in, 210
  management of, 219–221
  subarachnoid hemorrhage in,
    210–212
  symptoms, 213
Henle loop, 82
Heparin
  in deep venous thrombosis prophy-
    laxis, 108–109
  in ischemic stroke, 219
  low-molecular-weight
    in deep venous thrombosis pro-
      phylaxis, 109
    in ischemic stroke, 219
    in myocardial infarction, 121
    in venous thromboembolism,
      193
  in myocardial infarction, 121
  in parenteral nutrition, 101
  in venous thromboembolism,
    192–193
Heparin-induced thrombocytopenia,
  109, 193
Hepatitis, liver failure in, 175–176
Hepatorenal syndrome, 174, 181
Herpes simplex virus infection, acyclovir in, 184
Hespan, 66
Hetastarch, 66
Histamine-2 blockers
  in parenteral nutrition, 101
  in stress ulcer prophylaxis,
    110–111
Homans sign in deep venous thrombo-
  sis, 188
Hospital-acquired pneumonia,
  139–146
Hydralazine, 59

Hydrocephalus
  management in hemorrhagic
    strokes, 221
  in subarachnoid hemorrhage, 211
Hydrochloric acid in metabolic alkalosis, 89
Hydrochlorothiazide in heart failure,
  131
Hydrocortisone
  in acute respiratory distress syn-
    drome, 206
  dosage compared to other steroids,
    15t
  in sepsis, 155
Hypercalcemia, severe acute pancreatitis in, 160
Hypercapnia, permitted controlled in
  ARDS, 202–203
Hypercarbia from dead space, 26
Hypercoagulable states, 186
Hyperglycemia
  in cerebral vascular accident, 222
  from parenteral nutrition, 103
Hypertension
  intracerebral hemorrhage in, 210
  medications in, 58–59
Hyperthermia. *See* Fever
Hypertriglyceridemia
  from parenteral nutrition, 104
  severe acute pancreatitis in, 160
Hyperventilation in head injuries, 75
Hyponatremia in subarachnoid hemor-
  rhage, 211
Hypothermia in sepsis, 150
Hypovolemia, pulmonary artery cathe-
  ter measurements in, 52t
Hypovolemic shock, 11, 13
Hypoxia from shunts, 26

I
Imipenem
  in pneumonia, 145
  in severe acute pancreatitis, 168
Immune system in liver failure, 175,
  181
Inderal, 59
Infarction. *See* Myocardial infarction
Infectious agents
  in liver failure, 175–176
  in pneumonia, 141–142
  in sepsis, 151–152
  in severe acute pancreatitis, 161
Inferior vena cava filter in venous
    thromboembolism, 194–195
Inflammatory cascade
  in sepsis, 148
  in severe acute pancreatitis, 158–159

Inflammatory response syndrome, systemic (SIRS), 147–148
  in severe acute pancreatitis, 159
Inflection points in alveolar compliance curve, 35–36, 36f
Inotropes, 55–58, 56t
  in heart failure, 131
Inspiratory capacity, 30t
Inspiratory pressure, peak, 34–35, 35t
Inspiratory reserve volume, 30t
Insulin in parenteral nutrition, 101
Integrilin in myocardial infarction, 119
Interleukins (ILs)
  IL-1
    in sepsis, 148
    in severe acute pancreatitis, 158
  IL-6 in severe acute pancreatitis, 158
Intestinal mucosal atrophy in parenteral nutrition, 104
Intracranial pressure
  increased, 67–77
    diagnosis of, 68–69
    in hepatic encephalopathy, 173, 179
    and mean arterial pressure in head injury, 71–72, 72f
    monitoring in hemorrhagic stroke, 222
Intravascular coagulation, disseminated, in head injuries, 70
Intravenous fluids, crystalloid, 65t, 65–66
Intubation, indications for, 30–31
Inverse ratio ventilation in acute respiratory distress syndrome, 204–205
Ipratropium bromide in COPD, 136
  albuterol with, 136
Irbesartan in heart failure, 130
Ischemic attack, transient, 207–208
Ischemic stroke, 208–210
  blood pressure control in, 221
  embolic disease, 209–210
    radiographic tests in, 215–216
  management of, 216–219
  symptoms, 212
  thrombotic disease, 208–209
    large-vessel, 208
    small-vessel, 209
Isopropyl alcohol ingestion, osmolar gap from, 85
Isoproterenol, 56t, 57
Isuprel, 56t, 57

J
Jejunostomy tube, 95
Jugular venous oxygen saturation, internal, monitoring in head injuries, 75–76

K
Kidneys, 82–83
  failure of
    in liver failure, 174, 181
    in severe acute pancreatitis, 168
  renal tubular acidosis, 83–84
  in sepsis, 151, 154

L
Labetalol, 59
  in hypertension, 221, 222
β-Lactamase inhibitors in pneumonia, 145
Lactulose in hepatic encephalopathy, 179
Lasix in heart failure, 131
Left-to-right shunt, cardiac output measurement in, 49t
Left ventricle
  assist device in heart failure, 132
  diastolic and systolic pressures in cardiac cycle, 9f, 9–10
    and differential diagnosis of dysfunction, 10
  end diastolic pressure
    relation to end diastolic volume, 7f, 7–8
    relation to stroke volume, 8f, 8–9
  infarction, pulmonary artery catheter measurements in, 52t
  pressure rule of fives, 46t
Levaquin. See Levofloxacin
Levofloxacin
  in COPD, 136
  in pneumonia, 145
Levophed. See Norepinephrine
Lipase levels in severe acute pancreatitis, 164
Lipohyalinosis, ischemic strokes in, 209
Lisinopril in heart failure, 129
Liver
  acute fatty, of pregnancy, 184
  Budd-Chiari syndrome, 177, 183
  enzyme levels in severe acute pancreatitis, 164
  failure of, 171–184
    acetaminophen-induced, 176, 182, 183
    cardiovascular system in, 173, 180
    central nervous system in, 172–173, 179
    definition, 171–172
    diagnosis, 178
    gastrointestinal tract in, 174, 181
    hematologic disorders in, 175, 181–182
    immune system in, 175, 181
    management, 179–184

metabolic disorders in, 175, 182
pathophysiology, 172–175
possible etiologies, 175–177
pulmonary artery catheter measurements in, 52t
pulmonary disorders in, 173–174, 180
renal failure in, 174, 181
shock in, 12
symptoms and signs, 177–178
transplantation in, 182
hepatic encephalopathy, 172–173
management of, 179
transplantation of, 182
Loop of Henle, 82
Lopressor, 59
Lorazepam, 61
Losartan in heart failure, 130
Lovenox. *See* Enoxaparin
Löwenberg sign in deep venous thrombosis, 188
Lumbar puncture in strokes, 216
Lungs
chronic obstructive disease, 133–137. *See also* COPD (chronic obstructive pulmonary disease)
expiratory reserve volume, 30f
functional residual capacity, 30f
inspiratory capacity, 30f
inspiratory reserve volume, 30f
in liver failure, 173–174, 180
residual volume, 30f
tidal volume, 30f
total capacity, 30f
ventilator-induced injury, 199
vital capacity, 30f
volumes, 30f
West zones of, 27f, 27–28
pressure relationships in, 49t

M
Macrolides in pneumonia, 145
Magnesium in parenteral nutrition, 101t
Magnesium sulfate in hemorrhagic strokes, 220
Magnetic resonance imaging
cholangiopancreatography in severe acute pancreatitis, 165
in strokes, 214
venography in deep venous thrombosis, 190
Mannitol in head injuries, 73
Mean airway pressure (Map)
in acute respiratory distress syndrome, 203, 204
and arterial partial pressure of oxygen, 33f, 34, 41

Mean arterial pressure (MAP)
and cerebral perfusion pressure in head injury, 71–72, 72f
management in hemorrhagic stroke, 220
in sepsis, 151
Mechanical ventilation, 29–44
in acute respiratory distress syndrome, 201–205
inspired fraction of oxygen in, 201
inverse ratio in, 204–205
low tidal volume in, 202
permitted controlled hypercapnia in, 202–203
positive end-expiratory pressure in, 203–204
pressure control in, 204
volume control in, 204
assist control, 38–39, 39t
basic concepts of, 32–38
bi-level positive airway pressure, 40, 40t
in COPD, 135, 136, 137
goals of, 30
in heart failure, 128–129
increasing autoPEEP in, 38
and indications for intubation, 30–31
lung injury from, 199
measurement of pulmonary capillary wedge pressure in, 50, 50f
in myocardial infarction, 118
in pneumonia, 143
positive pressure modes, 38–41
pressure control, 40–41, 41t, 204
pressure support, 39–40, 40t
pressure *versus* volume control in, 41–42, 42f
in sepsis, 151
in severe acute pancreatitis, 166, 167
in strokes, 216
synchronized intermittent mandatory, 39, 39t
in venous thromboembolism, 192
weaning from, 42–44
Medications, 53–66. *See also* Drug-induced conditions
analgesics and sedatives, 60–61
anti-hypertensives, 58–59
blood products, 62–65
intravenous fluids, 65–66
paralytics, 62
pressors and inotropes, 55–58, 56t
receptors for, and mechanism of action, 54–55
Mefoxin in pneumonia, 145

Mental status
  in acute respiratory distress syndrome, 200
  in intracranial pressure increase, 68
Meropenem in pneumonia, 145
Merrem in pneumonia, 145
Metabolic acidosis, 80–81, 83–87
  clinical correlation, 86t, 86–87
  increased anion gap, 84–85
  normal anion gap, 83–84
  osmolar gap, 85–86
Metabolic alkalosis, 80–81, 87–89
  effects of alkalemia in, 88
  etiology of, 87–88
  treatment of, 88–89
Metabolic compensation, 81t
Metabolism
  basal rate estimation, 105
  disorders of
    in hemorrhagic stroke, 222
    liver failure in, 175, 177, 182
Methanol ingestion, osmolar gap from, 85
Methylprednisolone
  in acute respiratory distress syndrome, 206
  in COPD, 137
  dosage compared to other steroids, 15t
Metoclopramide in parenteral nutrition, 101
Metolazone in heart failure, 131
Metoprolol, 59
Metronidazole
  in pneumonia, 145
  severe acute pancreatitis from, 160
Midazolam, 61
Midodrine in liver failure, 181
Milrinone, 56t, 58
  in heart failure, 131
Minute volume, 24
Mnemonic for increased anion gap acidosis, 85t
Monro-Kellie hypothesis, 71
Morphine, 60
  in myocardial infarction, 120
Mu receptor, 55
MUDPILES mnemonic for increased anion gap acidosis, 85t
Multiple organ failure in sepsis, 149, 151
Myocardial infarction, 115–123
  airway management in, 118
  angiotensin-converting enzyme inhibitors in, 120
  aspirin in, 118
  beta-blockers in, 120
  definition, 115

  diagnosis, 117–118
  factors affecting severity, 116
  glycoprotein antagonists in, 119
  hemodynamic considerations in, 122–123
  heparin in, 121
  management, 118–123
  morphine in, 120
  nitrates in, 119, 120t
  order of events in, 116
  oxygenation in, 118
  revascularization options in, 121–122
  risk factors, 115–116
  symptoms and signs, 116–117
  thrombolytic therapy in, 121–122

N
Naloxone for opiate toxicity reversal, 60
Narcan for opiate toxicity reversal, 60
Nasoduodenal tube, 94–95
Nasogastric tube, 94
Nasojejunal tube, 95
Natrecor in heart failure, 131
Natriuretic peptides in heart failure, 127, 128
Necrosis, pancreatic, management of, 169
Neomycin in hepatic encephalopathy, 179
Neo-Synephrine. *See* Phenylephrine
Nephron function, 82–83
Nesiritide in heart failure, 131
Neurogenic shock, 11
Nimbex. *See* Cisatracurium
Nimodipine in subarachnoid hemorrhage, 220
Nimotop in subarachnoid hemorrhage, 220
Nipride. *See* Sodium nitroprusside
Nitrates in myocardial infarction, 119, 120t
Nitric oxide, inhaled
  in acute respiratory distress syndrome, 205
  in venous thromboembolism, 196
Nitrogen balance, assessment of, 105
Nitroglycerin, 58–59
  in heart failure, 131
  in hypertension, 221, 222
Nitroprusside. *See* Sodium nitroprusside
Norcuron, 62
Norepinephrine, 56, 56t
  in hypertension, 221, 222
  in liver failure, 180
  in sepsis, 154
  in severe acute pancreatitis, 167
  in venous thromboembolism, 195

Normodyne. *See* Labetalol
NovoSeven transfusions, 64
Nutrition, 93–105
 and assessing nutritional status, 105
 enteral, 93–99
 in hepatic encephalopathy, 179
 in liver failure, 182
 parenteral, 99–104
 in severe acute pancreatitis, 168–169

O
Octreotide in liver failure, 181
Ohm's law, 3
Opioids, 60
 toxicity reversal with naloxone, 60
Osmolar gap acidosis, 85–86
 clinical correlation, 86–87
 determination of, 85
 treatment of, 85–86
Osmolarity of formulas for tube feeding, 97
Oxygen
 alveolar-arterial diffusion gradient,
  19
  in pulmonary embolism, 191
 alveolar partial pressure, 19
 arterial content, 21
 arterial partial pressure, 19
  in acute respiratory distress syndrome, 200, 201
  and mean airway pressure, 33f,
   34, 42t
  normal, 80
  in pulmonary embolism, 191
  saturation related to, 20, 20f
  in sepsis, 151
 consumption per minute, 21
  pulmonary artery catheter measurements, 51t
  relation to delivery, 23, 23f
 delivery per minute, 21
  pulmonary artery catheter measurements, 51t
  relation to consumption, 23, 23f
 disassociation curve, 20
 extraction ratio, 21
  pulmonary artery catheter measurements, 51t
 inspired fraction, 19
  in acute respiratory distress syndrome, 200, 201
  in sepsis, 151
  in severe acute pancreatitis, 167
  in venous thromboembolism, 192
 mixed venous oxygen saturation,
  pulmonary artery catheter
  measurements of, 51t, 52t

partial pressure
 alveolar, 19
 arterial, 19
 derivation of, 18–20
 ideal value, 18, 24
 inspired, 19
Oxygenation, 18–24
 in acute respiratory distress syndrome, 201
 in COPD, 135–136
 in heart failure, 129
 in liver failure, 180
 in myocardial infarction, 118
 in pneumonia, 143
 in sepsis, 151
 in severe acute pancreatitis, 167
 in venous thromboembolism, 192

P
Pacing, biventricular, in heart failure, 132
Pain
 in myocardial infarction, 117
 in severe acute pancreatitis, 162–163
Palla sign in pulmonary embolism, 191
Pancreas divisum, 161–162
Pancreatitis, severe acute, 157–170
 airway management, 166
 alcohol-induced, 159–160
 amylase levels in, 163–164
 antimicrobial therapy in, 168
 cardiovascular support in, 167–168
 in cystic fibrosis, 162
 deep venous thrombosis prophylaxis in, 170
 definition, 157–158
 diagnosis, 163–166
 drug-induced, 160
 in gallstone disease, 159, 169–170
 glucose levels in, 168
 in hypercalcemia, 160
 in hypertriglyceridemia, 160
 idiopathic, 162
 in infections, 161
 inflammatory cascade in, 158–159
 laboratory tests in, 163–164
 lipase levels in, 164
 liver enzymes in, 164
 localized to pancreas, 158
 management, 166–170
 necrosis management in, 169
 nutrition in, 168–169
 in pancreas divisum, 161–162
 pathophysiology, 158–159
 possible etiologies, 159–161
 post-endoscopic retrograde cholangiopancreatography, 162
 in pregnancy, 162

radiographic tests in, 164–166
renal failure in, 168
scoring of severity, 166
stress ulcer prophylaxis in, 170
supportive management, 167
symptoms and signs of, 162–163
systemic response in, 159
in trauma, 161
in vascular disease, 162
Papaverine, intra-arterial, in vasospasm, 221
Paracetamol, liver failure from, 176, 182
Paralytic agents, 62
in head injuries, 76
Parenteral nutrition, 99–104
additives in, 101–102
carbohydrates in, 100
clinical correlation, 102–103
composition of, 99–102
electrolyte abnormalities in, 103–104
electrolytes in, 101, 101t
fats in, 100–101
gut changes from, 103–104
hyperglycemia in, 103–104
hypertriglyceridemia in, 104
indications for, 99
potential complications of, 103–104
central line-related, 104
protein in, 99–100
Peak inspiratory pressure, 34–35, 35t
Peak to pause pressures, 34–35, 35t
PEEP. *See* Positive end-expiratory pressure (PEEP)
Pentamidine, severe acute pancreatitis
from, 160
Pentobarbital coma in head injuries,
76–77
Perfusion mismatch with ventilation,
26–27
in pulmonary embolism, 191, 191t
Persantine in ischemic stroke, 219
pH
in acidemia, 80
in acidosis, 80t
in alkalemia, 80
in alkalosis, 80t
ideal value, 18, 24
normal, 80
Phenylephrine, 55–56, 56t
in hypertension, 221, 222
in liver failure, 180
in sepsis, 154
in severe acute pancreatitis, 168
in venous thromboembolism, 195
Phlegmasia
alba dolens, 186
cerulea dolens, 186

Phosphodiesterase inhibitors, 56t, 58
in heart failure, 131
in myocardial infarction, 123
Phosphorus in parenteral nutrition, 101t
Pink puffer, 133
Piperacillin/tazobactam in pneumonia,
145
Plasma, fresh frozen, 64
Plateau pressure, 34–35, 35t
Platelets
antiplatelet medications in ischemic
stroke, 218
transfusions of, 63
in liver failure, 181
Plavix in ischemic stroke, 219
Plethysmography, impedance, in deep
venous thrombosis, 190
Pneumonia, 139–146
airway management in, 143
antimicrobial therapy in, 144–146
dosages of, 145–146
duration of, 145
community-acquired, 139–146
antimicrobial therapy, 144
definition, 139
microbiology, 141
pathophysiology, 140–141
diagnosis, 142–143
hospital-acquired, 139–146
antimicrobial therapy, 144
definition, 139
microbiology, 141–142
pathophysiology, 140–141
mechanical ventilation in, 143
oxygenation in, 143
symptoms and signs, 142
treatment, 143–146
Positioning
of head, in head injuries, 72–73
prone, in acute respiratory distress
syndrome, 205
Positive end-expiratory pressure
(PEEP), 35–37
in acute respiratory distress syndrome, 203–204
affecting pulmonary capillary
wedge pressure, 51
and autoPEEP, 37–38
goals of, 36
in liver failure, 180
Positive pressure in COPD, noninvasive, 136, 137
Potassium in parenteral nutrition, 101t
Precedex, 61
Prednisone
in COPD, 137
dosage compared to other steroids, 15t

Pregnancy
    acute fatty liver of, 184
    severe acute pancreatitis in, 162
Pressors and inotropes, 55–58, 56t
Pressure control ventilation, 40–41, 41t
    in acute respiratory distress syn-
        drome, 204
    compared to volume control, 41–42,
        42f, 42t
Pressure support ventilation, 39–40, 40t
    weaning from, 44
Primacor. See Milrinone
Primaxin in pneumonia, 145
ProAmatine in liver failure, 181
Prone positioning in acute respiratory
    distress syndrome, 205
Prophylaxis
    against deep venous thrombosis,
        107–109
    against stress ulceration, 110–111
Propofol, 61
Propranolol, 59
Protein in parenteral nutrition,
    99–100
Protein C, activated, in sepsis, 149,
    155–156
Proton pump inhibitor in stress ulcer
    prophylaxis, 111
Pulmonary artery catheters (Swan-
    Ganz), 45–52
    clinical correlation, 52, 52t
    common measurements, 51t
    measurements in various conditions,
        52t
    in venous thromboembolism, 195
Pulmonary artery pressure
    in lung zones, 49t
    normal, 46t, 47
    rule of fives, 46t
    wedge pressure in acute respiratory
        distress syndrome, 197
Pulmonary capillary wedge pressure,
    49–52
    autoPEEP affecting, 51
    at end expiration, 50, 50f
    as estimate of preload, 49
    in lung zones, 49t, 49–50
    in mechanical ventilation, 50, 50f
    normal pressure, 46t, 47
    PEEP affecting, 51
    pressure rule of fives, 46t
    respiratory variation in, 50, 50f
    in spontaneous breathing, 50, 50f
    in venous thromboembolism, 195
    and volume status assessment, 49
Pulmonary embolism, 186, 187
    diagnosis, 190–192, 191t

    embolectomy, 196
    pulmonary artery catheter measure-
        ments in, 52t
    symptoms and signs, 187–188
Pulmonary system
    chronic obstructive disease, 133–137.
        See also COPD (chronic
        obstructive pulmonary disease)
    response in shock, 12
Pulmonary vascular resistance
    index in pulmonary artery catheter
        measurements, 51t
    in pulmonary embolism, 187
Pupillary responses in intracranial
    pressure increase, 68

R
Radiography
    in liver failure, 178
    in placement of feeding tubes, 96
    in severe acute pancreatitis,
        164–166
Rebleeding in subarachnoid hemor-
    rhage, 212
Receptors for medications, 54–55
Refeeding syndrome in parenteral
    nutrition, 104
Reglan in parenteral nutrition, 101
Renal function, 82–83. See also Kidneys
ReoPro in myocardial infarction, 119
Reserve volumes, expiratory and
    inspiratory, 30t
Residual capacity, functional
    and closing volume, 32f, 32–33
    prone positioning affecting, 205
Respiratory acidosis, 80–81, 89–90
    treatment, 90
Respiratory alkalosis, 80–81, 90–91
    treatment, 91
Respiratory compensation, 81t
Respiratory distress, 197–206. See also
    Acute respiratory distress syn-
    drome (ARDS)
Respiratory failure
    hypoxic, 30–31
    intubation in, 30–31
    peri-operative, 31
    in shock, 31
    ventilatory, 31
Respiratory quotient, 25
    dietary intake affecting, 105
Respiratory rate, 24
Respiratory system in sepsis, 151
Retavase in myocardial infarction, 121
Reteplase in myocardial infarction, 121
Revascularization options in myocar-
    dial infarction, 121–122

Right atrial pressure
  and cardiac output, 6–7, 7f
  normal, 46t, 47
  rule of fives, 46t
Right-to-left shunt, cardiac output measurement in, 49t
Right ventricle
  infarction, pulmonary artery catheter measurements in, 52t
  normal pressure, 46t, 47
  pressure rule of fives, 46t
Ringer's solution, 65–66
Rocephin in pneumonia, 145
Rule of fives, 46t

S
Salicylates, severe acute pancreatitis from, 160
Saline solutions, 65–66
Salt wasting, cerebral
  in cerebral vascular accident, 222
  in head injuries, 70
Sandostatin in liver failure, 181
Scintigraphy in pulmonary embolism, 191, 191t
Sedation in head injuries, 76
Sedatives and analgesics, 60–62
Seizures in subarachnoid hemorrhage, 212
Sepsis, 147–156
  acute respiratory distress syndrome in, 154
  airway management in, 151
  antifungal therapy in, 152–153
  antimicrobial therapy in, 151–152
  cardiovascular support in, 153–154
  deep venous thrombosis prophylaxis in, 156
  definitions, 147–148
  diagnosis, 150–151
  glucose levels in, 154
  infection control in, 153
  in liver failure, 175
  management, 151–156
  nutrition in, 154
  oxygenation in, 151
  pathophysiology, 148–149
  pulmonary artery catheter measurements in, 52t
  recombinant human activated protein C in, 155–156
  renal failure in, 151, 154
  steroid therapy in, 154–155
  stress ulcer prophylaxis in, 156
  symptoms and signs, 149–150
Septic shock, 11, 13, 148

Shock, 11–15
  in adrenal insufficiency, 12
    treatment of, 15
  anaphylactic, 12
    treatment of, 15
  cardiac output in, 12, 13, 13t
  cardiogenic, 11, 13
    treatment of, 13–14
  hypovolemic, 11, 13
    treatment of, 14
  in liver failure, 12
    treatment of, 15
  neurogenic, 12
    treatment of, 14–15
  organ systems in, 12
  respiratory failure in, 31
  septic, 11, 13, 148
    treatment of, 14
  treatment of, 13–15, 15t
  types of, 11–12
Shohl solution in renal tubular acidosis, 84
Shunts
  cardiac output measurements in, 49t
  causes of, 26
  hypoxia in, 26
  in pulmonary embolism, 187
Skin response in shock, 12
Sodium
  hyponatremia in subarachnoid hemorrhage, 211
  in parenteral nutrition, 101t
Sodium nitroprusside, 58
  in heart failure, 131
  in hypertension, 221, 222
  intrathecal, in vasospasm, 221
Solu-Cortef in sepsis, 155
Solu-Medrol. See Methylprednisolone
Spirometry in COPD, 135
Spironolactone in heart failure, 130
Sputum in pneumonia, 142–143
Starling curve, 8f, 8–9
Steroid therapy
  in acute respiratory distress syndrome, 206
  in COPD, 137
  equivalent doses in, 15t
  in sepsis, 154–155
Streptase. See Streptokinase
Streptokinase
  in myocardial infarction, 122
  in venous thromboembolism, 196
Stress ulcer prophylaxis, 110–111
  in cerebral vascular accident, 222
  in liver failure, 181
  in sepsis, 156
  in severe acute pancreatitis, 170

Stroke, 207–223. *See also* Cerebral vascular accident
Stroke volume
  index measurements with pulmonary artery catheter, 51t
  and left ventricular end diastolic pressure, 8f, 8–9
Subarachnoid hemorrhage
  management of, 219–221
  strokes in, 210–212
Sucralfate in stress ulcer prophylaxis, 110
Sulfasalazine, severe acute pancreatitis from, 160
Sulfonamides, severe acute pancreatitis from, 160
Sulindac, severe acute pancreatitis from, 160
Surgery
  deep venous thrombosis prophylaxis in, 107
  in intracranial aneurysms, 219
  in placement of feeding tubes, 97
Swallowing function evaluation before oral feeding, 222
Swan-Ganz catheters, 45–52. *See also* Pulmonary artery catheters (Swan-Ganz)
Sympathetic nervous system in heart failure, 126
Synchronized intermittent mandatory ventilation, 39, 39t
  weaning from, 44
Systemic inflammatory response syndrome (SIRS), 147–148
  in severe acute pancreatitis, 159
Systemic vascular resistance
  equation for, 46
  pulmonary artery catheter measurements, 51t

T
Tamoxifen, severe acute pancreatitis from, 161
Tamponade, cardiac, pulmonary artery catheter measurements in, 52t
Temperature
  hyperthermia. *See* Fever
  hypothermia in sepsis, 150
  maintenance of
    in cerebral vascular accident, 222
    in head injuries, 74
Tetracycline, severe acute pancreatitis from, 160
Thermodilution technique for cardiac output measurement, 48–49
  potential errors in, 49, 49t

Thiazides
  in heart failure, 131
  severe acute pancreatitis from, 160
Thrombocytopenia, heparin-induced, 109, 193
Thromboembolism, venous, 185–196
  cardiovascular support in, 195
  and deep venous thrombosis, 186
  definition, 185–186
  diagnosis, 188–192
    in deep venous thrombosis, 188–190
    in pulmonary embolism, 190–192, 191t
  heparin in, 192–193
    low-molecular-weight heparin, 193
  inferior vena cava filter in, 194–195
  management of, 192–196
    duration of anticoagulation therapy in, 194
  pathophysiology, 186–187
  and pulmonary embolism, 187
  symptoms and signs, 187–188
  vasopressor therapy in, 195
  warfarin in, 193–194
Thrombolytic therapy
  contraindications, 217
  in ischemic stroke, 216–218
  in myocardial infarction, 121–122
  in venous thromboembolism, 196
Thrombophilic disorders, deep venous thrombosis prophylaxis in, 107–108
Thrombophlebitis in deep venous thrombosis, 186
Thrombosis, deep venous
  diagnosis, 188–190
  pathophysiology, 186
  prophylaxis
    in sepsis, 156
    in severe acute pancreatitis, 170
  risk factors, 107–108
  symptoms and signs, 187, 188
  and thromboembolism, 185
  treatment options, 108–109
Thrombotic disease, ischemic stroke in, 208–209. *See also* Ischemic stroke, thrombotic disease
Thrombus, catheter, cardiac output measurement in, 49t
Ticlid. *See* Ticlopidine
Ticlopidine
  in ischemic stroke, 219
  in myocardial infarction, 119

Tidal volume, 24, 30t
  low tidal volume ventilation in
    ARDS, 202
Tirofiban in myocardial infarction,
  119
Tissue cultures in pneumonia, 143
Torsemide in heart failure, 131
Total lung capacity, 30f
  and functional residual capacity, 32
t-PA. *See* Alteplase
Tracheobronchial aspirate in pneumo-
  nia, 143
Transfusions. *See* Blood, products
Transient ischemic attack, 207–208
Transplantation of liver, 182
Trauma
  head injuries, 67–77
  severe acute pancreatitis from, 161
Tricuspid insufficiency, cardiac output
    measurement in, 49t
Triglyceride levels
  in parenteral feeding, 104
  in severe acute pancreatitis, 160
Triple-H therapy in hemorrhagic
    strokes, 220
Troponin I levels in myocardial infarc-
  tion, 118t
Trypsin in severe acute pancreatitis,
  158
Tube feeding. *See* Enteral nutrition
Tubules, renal, 82–83
Tumor necrosis factor-α
  in sepsis, 148
  in severe acute pancreatitis, 158

U
Ulcers, stress, prophylaxis against,
  110–111
Ultrasonography
  in deep venous thrombosis, 189
  in liver failure, 178
  in severe acute pancreatitis, 165
  in strokes, 215, 216
Unasyn in pneumonia, 145
Urine output in sepsis, 151

V
Valproic acid, severe acute pancreatitis
  from, 160
Valsartan in heart failure, 130
Vancocin in pneumonia, 145–146
Vancomycin in pneumonia, 145–146
Vascular disorders
  coronary arteries in myocardial
    infarction, 116
  liver failure in, 177
  severe acute pancreatitis in, 162

Vascular resistance
  pulmonary
    index measurements with pulmo-
      nary artery catheter, 51t
    in pulmonary embolism, 187
  systemic
    equation for, 46
    pulmonary artery catheter mea-
      surements, 51t
Vasoconstriction, and cardiac output, 5
Vasodilatation, and cardiac output, 5
Vasodilators in heart failure, 131
Vasopressin, 56t, 58
  in liver failure, 180
  in sepsis, 154
  in severe acute pancreatitis, 167, 168
  in venous thromboembolism, 195
Vasopressor therapy
  in liver failure, 180
  in sepsis, 153–154
  in severe acute pancreatitis, 167–168
  in venous thromboembolism, 195
Vasospasm
  management in hemorrhagic
    strokes, 220–221
  in subarachnoid hemorrhage, 211
Vasotec in heart failure, 129
Vecuronium, 62
Vena cava, inferior, filter in venous
    thromboembolism, 194–195
Venography in deep venous thrombosis
  contrast, 189
  magnetic resonance, 190
Venous pressure. *See* Central venous
    pressure
Venous return, and cardiac output, 6–7,
  7f
Venous thromboembolism, 185–196
Venous thrombosis, 185, 186
Ventilation, 24–28
  mechanical, 29–44. *See also* Mechani-
    cal ventilation
Ventilation/perfusion matching
  inhaled nitric oxide affecting, 205
  prone positioning affecting, 205
Ventilation/perfusion mismatch, 26–27
  in pulmonary embolism, 191, 191t
Ventilator-induced lung injury, 199. *See
    also* Mechanical ventilation
Ventolin. *See* Albuterol in COPD
Ventricular function. *See* Left ventricle;
    Right ventricle
  and cardiac output, 3–10
Ventriculostomy drain
  in head injuries, 69
  in hemorrhagic strokes, 221

Versed, 61
Virchow triad in deep venous thrombosis, 186
Vital capacity, 30t
Vitamin K in parenteral nutrition, 102
Volume control ventilation
    in acute respiratory distress syndrome, 204
    compared to pressure contro, 41–42, 42fl, 42t
Volume status of patient, and pulmonary capillary wedge pressure, 49
Volumes, lung, 30f

W
Warfarin
    in deep venous thrombosis prophylaxis, 109
    in venous thromboembolism, 193–194
Waveforms
    central venous pressure, 47f
    "floating swan," 48f

Weaning from ventilator, 42–44
    continuous positive airway pressure in, 43–44
    pressure support wean in, 44
    synchronous intermittent mandatory wean in, 44
West zones of lung, 27f, 27–28
    pressure relationships in, 49t
Westermark sign in pulmonary embolism, 191
White cell count in sepsis, 150, 151

X
Xigris in sepsis, 155

Z
Zaroxolyn in heart failure, 131
Zestril in heart failure, 129
Zinc in parenteral nutrition, 101
Zithromax in pneumonia, 145
Zosyn in pneumonia, 145
Zovirax in herpes simplex virus infection, 184